WLS
WILDERNESS LIFE SUPPORT

PREVENTION • DIAGNOSIS • TREATMENT • EVACUATION

A Text for Wilderness First Aid Courses

SENIOR EDITOR
DAVID DELLA-GIUSTINA MD, FAWM
ASSOCIATE PROFESSOR
EMERGENCY MEDICINE RESIDENCY PROGRAM DIRECTOR
WILDERNESS FELLOWSHIP PROGRAM DIRECTOR
CHIEF, SECTION OF EDUCATION
DEPARTMENT OF EMERGENCY MEDICINE
YALE SCHOOL OF MEDICINE

EDITORS
RICHARD INGEBRETSEN MD, PHD
CLINICAL INSTRUCTOR OF MEDICINE
UNIVERSITY OF UTAH SCHOOL OF MEDICINE

STEVEN ROY MD, NR-EMT, FAWN, DIMM
MCGILL UNIVERSITY

ILLUSTRATIONS
MICHAEL DIDIER

Edition 2.0

© 2018 by Travel Medicine Press
ISBN: 978-0-692-19341-9

Previous edition published in 2015 under ISBN 978-0-578-15338-4

All Rights Reserved. No part of this book may be reproduced in any manner without the express written consent of the authors with the exception of images referenced below.

Permission is granted to copy, distribute and/or modify the following images: 4.1, 14.1 under the terms of the GNU Free Documentation License, Version 1.1 or any later version published by the Free Software Foundation; with no Invariant Sections, no Front-Cover Texts, and no Back-Cover Texts.

TABLE OF CONTENTS

Chapter 1:	Patient Assessment	1
Chapter 2:	Vital Sign Assessment	14
Chapter 3:	Airway and Breathing	19
Chapter 4:	Bleeding and Shock	25
Chapter 5:	Abdominal and Chest Injuries	31
Chapter 6:	Musculoskeletal Injuries	38
Chapter 7:	Drowning and Water Safety	47
Chapter 8:	Lightning Injuries and Prevention	52
Chapter 9:	Head Trauma and Spine Injuries	59
Chapter 10:	Medical Problems in the Wilderness	66
Chapter 11:	Wilderness Wound Management	78
Chapter 12:	Heat Induced Injuries	90
Chapter 13:	Hypothermia and Cold Injuries	98
Chapter 14:	Bites and Stings	105
Chapter 15:	Evacuation Guidelines	119
Chapter 16:	Wilderness Medical Kits	124
Chapter 17:	Water Disinfection and Hydration	129
Acronyms		137
Glossary of Terms		139
Improvised Litters		147
SOAP Note		149

CHAPTER 1

Patient Assessment

Objectives:
- Recognize possible threats to rescuer(s) and patient(s) and identify resources by adequately surveying the scene.
- Rapidly detect any immediately life-threatening conditions while making appropriate interventions during the primary survey.
- Obtain a thorough history and perform an appropriate physical exam as part of the secondary survey.
- Describe the unique components of the ongoing survey in a wilderness environment.
- Understand the importance of the following acronyms in pre-hospital patient care: MARCH, CARTS, AVPU, SAMPLE, COLDERR and C-SPINE.

Overview

- You are being trained to be a first responder in a wilderness emergency medical situation. These situations may be confusing and emotionally charged.
- The purpose of this chapter is to help you to develop a process that will allow you to overcome obstacles and provide the patient(s) with the appropriate care.

Scene Survey

- Responders should begin each rescue by surveying the scene.
- The scene survey consists of several parts, but the most important is safety for you, other rescuers and the victims. Placing a rescuer at undue risk can complicate the situation, if not create additional patients. We do not want to create another victim.
- Surveying the scene requires you to identify the number of patients; have an understanding of each patient's condition; and note the presence of bystanders, equipment, and other clues that may be useful in determining the cause of the injury or illness.

Scene Safety

- Is the scene safe for me to enter? Consider external hazards such as the following:
  - Physical dangers (rocks, snow/ice, trees, fires, wildlife, etc.)
  - Weather/environment (hot/cold temperatures, lightning, high altitude, etc.)
  - Other people (bikers on single track, climbers above you, hunters, etc.)
- Will the scene remain safe? If not, what is my plan?
  - Safe zones
  - Moving patients to a safe area
- Is it safe for me to physically care for the patient(s)? Gloves and barrier devices, such as a face mask, should be considered with every patient to prevent disease transmission through bleeding, vomiting, etc.
- How many patients are there? Which one(s) need help first?
  - The victim's equipment may provide information about the mechanism of injury (MOI).
  - Bystanders may have witnessed the victim's injury or may be able to assist with patient care.
- Are there resources near the scene that may be useful in treating or evacuating the patient?

Approaching, Identifying, and Getting Permission to Treat the Victim(s)

- When approaching the victim, use caution so that you do not expose them to additional hazards such as rock or icefall. Consider marking the route to the scene if additional rescuers are to follow.
- Immediately identify yourself and request the victim's permission to treat. If the victim is unconscious or confused, then their consent to treatment is implied. Otherwise, the victim has the right to decline treatment.
- Ask the victim's name and say "can you tell me what happened?" If the patient cannot answer these questions, they are either unconscious or have an altered level of responsiveness; start with the primary survey.
- This is an opportunity to determine the Level of Consciousness (LOC) of your patient. For this we use the **AVPU** (Alert, Verbal Painful, Unresponsive) scale. Is the patient **A**lert and oriented, responsive only to **V**erbal stimulation (talking to them), responsive only to **P**ainful stimulation, or **U**nresponsive to any stimulation? If the victim shows any signs of life such as movement, moaning, or talking, then you move on to the primary survey (below). For those victims who are completely unresponsive, the rescuer must quickly move forward with Basic Life Support (BLS) / CPR. This is extremely important if the situation involves a lightning strike, drowning or avalanche. These are wilderness situations where immediate CPR, which includes breathing for the victim, may save a victim's life.

Primary Survey: Disability
Level of Responsiveness

A   Alert
V   Verbal – Awakens briefly, withdraws, or moans when spoken to
P   Pain – Awakens briefly, withdraws, or moans in response to painful stimuli
U   Unresponsive – No response to any stimuli

Patient Assessment

The patient assessment is broken down into 4 parts:
- Primary Survey
- Secondary Survey
- Ongoing Survey
- Documentation

The urgency of these parts of the patient assessment decreases from primary survey to documentation. In the wilderness, complete documentation is really only necessary for complex patients.

Primary Survey

Primary Survey: MARCH

The goal of the Primary Survey is to identify and treat conditions that pose an immediate threat to life. Approaching the victim using the acronym **M A R C H** allows the rescuer to address the life-threatening issues in order of importance. Anytime there is major bleeding you should always **stop the bleeding**. Preventing major hemorrhage is so important that it supersedes airway in the acronym for the primary assessment - **M A R C H**. We are not able to replace massive blood loss in the wilderness, so we must do our best to preserve blood volume and our patients. Airway does come early in the MARCH acronym but massive hemorrhage is first. Therefore, we would stop the massive bleed before moving onto the airway. Evaluating the patient's pulses falls under the C for circulation in the MARCH acronym and would therefore not be the next best step.

Asking the patient if he takes any blood thinners will be part of your focused history, which comes after your primary assessment. You may be able to obtain this information during the primary assessment, but this should not distract from your assessment.

Because this portion of the assessment is searching for critical conditions, it is most applicable to patients who have an altered level of consciousness or have a significant injury. However, this survey should be utilized in *every* victim whom one treats in the wilderness. In those victims who are alert and appear well, this assessment may be brief. Problems found on the primary survey that are life threatening should be addressed immediately, before continuing the survey

Primary Survey:

M	Massive hemorrhage management
A	Airway with cervical spine stabilization
R	Respiration
C	Circulation
H	Hypothermia / Hyperthermia and Hike vs. Helicopter

M – Massive hemorrhage management
- The first objective is to stop massive hemorrhage rapidly because a victim can lose most of their blood volume in a matter of minutes with major arterial or venous bleeding.
- In the wilderness, you cannot replace this blood, and the victim may be required to be much more active than the typical hospitalized patient.
- This step is applicable only for major bleeding and does not include injuries with only minor oozing that will be addressed later in the secondary survey. Generally, these types of injuries are rare in the wilderness but can have fatal consequences if not treated rapidly.
- Treatment usually consists of the placement of a tourniquet if it is an extremity injury. If one does not have a tourniquet or if the injury is not amenable to the use of a tourniquet (e.g. facial or torso wound), then a pressure dressing directly on the area of bleeding is the best option.
- The placement of the tourniquet does not mandate that the tourniquet stay in place until the patient reaches definitive medical care. The expectation is that that the rescuer will reassess the wound and the bleeding after the patient has been stabilized in the secondary survey and ongoing assessment stage. The use of tourniquets and their management is covered in depth in the wound management chapter.

A – Airway with cervical spine stabilization
- The "airway" is the continuous path from the patient's lips all the way down to their vocal cords at the base of their throat. Any blockage of this pathway can limit the flow of air into the lungs.
- There are two issues in the assessment of the victim's airway:
  1. Is the airway currently open and is air flowing easily in and out?
  2. Is the victim able to keep their airway open with good air flow without your help? This is termed "maintaining their airway".
- First, Is the airway open?
  - If the awake victim is moving air but has noisy breathing, they will often put themselves in the best position that allows them to keep their airway open. Do not force them into a position that they do not want to go into. Generally, we like to place victims on their back, but you should not force a victim to this position if they cannot tolerate it.
  - If the victim has a decreased level of consciousness, then roll them onto their back as a single unit, being careful not to twist or jerk the spine or neck. Once the victim is on their back, then attempt to open the airway using the **head tilt-chin lift** maneuver (Figure 1.1) unless you think the victim was injured or involved in an accident.
  - If you suspect that the victim has head or spinal injuries, use the **jaw-thrust** technique to minimize neck movement by placing one hand on each side of the victim's head and grasping the angles of the victim's lower jaw and lifting up and forward with both hands (Figure 1.2).
  - If the victim has a decreased level of consciousness and is not moving air well with initial positioning, then inspect for and remove any foreign objects from their mouth. In victims of avalanches, snow burial, or major trauma, it is not unusual to see snow, teeth, dirt, and leaves in their mouths.
- Second, Is the victim able to maintain their airway?
  - There are potential airway issues, especially in trauma and allergic reactions, where the patient may develop worsening obstruction or blockage to their airway and have difficulty breathing. This is important when you consider how to evacuate the victim(s) and which victim should be evacuated first.

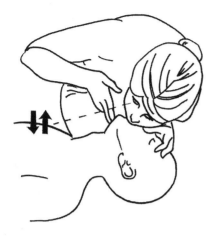

Figure 1.1 Head tilt chin lift   *Figure 1.2 Jaw thrust*

R – Respiration
- Respiration involves the evaluation of how well the patient is breathing and whether there is any potential for respiratory compromise in the future.
- If the victim does not start breathing after the airway has been opened, begin rescue breathing as described for basic CPR using current guidelines.
    - Each breath should be delivered over one second with enough air to see the chest rise.
    - If the breath does not go in, reposition the airway and try again.
- If the victim is breathing, briefly assess the quality of the respirations. Does the patient appear to be working hard to breathe, are they breathing rapidly/slowly, is their breathing appropriate, etc.?

C – Circulation
- Any patient who is awake or showing any sign of life will have a heartbeat. This step is to assess the victim's cardiovascular status with a focus on the heart rate, pulse strength and to treat non-massive hemorrhage.
- You can assess the pulse at the pedal/tibial, radial, brachial, femoral or carotid arteries.
    - Assess the quality of the pulse. Is it weak/thready, bounding, rapid, or irregular?
    - Check for bleeding by performing a blood sweep. This is a rapid (5 - 10 seconds) full, head-to-toe check for blood, wet clothing, swelling or other signs of significant bleeding.
- A blood sweep also affords the rescuer the opportunity to simultaneously note major deformities.

H – Hypothermia / Hyperthermia and Hike vs Helicopter
- At this point in the primary survey, the rescuer has treated any immediate threats to the patient's life and has taken steps to mitigate those threats. Wilderness medicine presents an additional issue that one must consider: the environment and its potential to worsen the victim's medical course.
- Recognize that whatever the environment, the victim has likely been exposed to it for a longer period and has not been compensating as well as the rescuers.
- A victim in a cold/hot environment will likely be colder/hotter than the rescuer.
- Steps should be taken to limit the victim's exposure to the environment.
- Hypothermia in trauma can lead to the cascade of acidosis and coagulopathy with increased mortality.
- Think about the evacuation plan (hike vs. helicopter).
    - The life-threatening injuries have been identified at this point.
    - What types of resources will you need and how can you get them to you to help your victims?
    - This is also a point to consider sending someone to go get help depending on the situation. This can be helpful because that individual can relay more valuable information beyond the initial "someone's unconscious."
    - If you are going to send somebody ahead to get help, you should send two people to help ensure that help is reached and that something does not occur to that single person sent out.

- As a general rule, especially when dealing with possible injuries to the spinal column, perform first aid on the victim where he or she lies. However, there are special circumstances under which there is potential for more severe injury or death if the victim is not moved.
- At the end of your primary survey, it is also the time to decide if this patient needs an immediate evacuation ("load and go") or if it's suitable to "stay and play" and to manage their issues at the current location.

Primary Survey in Conscious Patients
- When the patient is conscious, the rescuer may be able to substitute portions of the complete primary survey with questions. For example:
    - A talking patient has, for the time being, intact airway, breathing and circulation. The rescuer should still assess the quality of the breathing and pulse.
    - Asking a patient about what happened and if they are bleeding may eliminate the need for a blood sweep and spinal immobilization.

CPR – Cardiopulmonary Resuscitation

CPR Guideline Update
- The latest American Heart Association guidelines emphasize chest compressions during CPR by re-ordering the initial A-B-C to C-A-B and stating compressions should occur within the first 10 seconds of patient contact.
- The rescuer is advised to only briefly (5-10 seconds) check for signs of movement or breathing.
- The compression rate remains 100 per minute with a 30:2 compression-to-breath ratio for adult one- and two-rescuer as well as child/infant single-rescuer.
- Two-rescuer CPR for children/infants should be done at a 15:2 compression-to-breath ratio.
- The lay rescuer may provide "hands-only CPR" where no rescue breaths are delivered.
- Hand positioning remains in the center of the patient's sternum (chest), with a greater emphasis on ensuring adequate compression depth of at least two inches in adult patients and at least one-third of the depth of the patient's chest in children/infants.

Wilderness CPR Considerations
- CPR without rapid access to advanced medical care is unlikely to be successful.
- Do not start CPR in patients who have obvious signs of death such as rigor mortis or decapitation.
- CPR is exhausting to a rescuer, particularly in extreme conditions where energy may be required for self-evacuation. Safety of the rescuers should be considered in decisions regarding duration of CPR in the backcountry.
- If a patient has been pulseless for longer than 15 minutes, with or without CPR, further attempts at resuscitation should not be made (exceptions are lightning or hypothermia victims).
- A hypothermic patient is "not dead until warm and dead.". This means that a victim of cold exposure with hypothermia (low body temperature) should be evacuated and warmed up by medical personnel before declaring them dead. These victims may regain signs of life with warming.

Secondary Survey

The goal of the secondary survey is to identify and treat any remaining injuries and illnesses. These conditions may become problems if left unnoticed or if they require advanced medical attention. This portion of the patient assessment is comprised of two key elements:
- An abbreviated medical history
- A physical exam including vital signs

The order in which these components are performed depends on the issue. For example, a fallen rock climber should have the physical exam portion of the secondary survey performed first to identify any other traumatic injuries, whereas an abbreviated history from a camper who has developed abdominal pain may be more useful.

Abbreviated History

- Most of the patient's history is obtained immediately by asking "what happened?" However, a few other key questions must be answered to ensure the victim's problems are treated properly.
- The mnemonic **SAMPLE** will help you to remember the essential points of a patient history.
- For critical patients, you may be the only person who gets to talk to the patient while they are still conscious. Therefore, if an initially unconscious patient regains consciousness, immediately obtain a history.
- In patients with an altered level of consciousness, other clues may be needed to obtain the history. The mnemonic **AEIOUTIPS** can be helpful in unresponsive patients. A few examples of clues:
  - Medical alert tags can be found in the form of necklaces, bracelets, anklets, tattoos, etc.
  - List of medications or medical problems may be found in a wallet.
  - Medications or devices such as a glucometer (blood sugar meter) or epinephrine auto-injector may be found in a victim's bag/tent/pocket/etc.
  - Bystanders or family members may be familiar with a victim's past or present medical history.
  - Cell phones may be employed to contact family members.
- To assist you in characterizing a victim's pain, use the acronym **COLDERR**. Notice that this is most helpful in patients with pain from medical problems rather than traumatic injuries.

Secondary Survey: A Brief History

S	Signs and Symptoms (chief complaint)
A	Allergies – to anything
M	Medications/ Medical alert tags
P	Past medical / surgical history (illness and injuries)
L	Last meal
E	Events leading up to and causing the accident / injury (what happened?)

Formulating the Assessment: Altered Mental Status Patients

A	Allergies (anaphylaxis) / Altitude
E	Environment (hyper or hypothermia) / Epilepsy (seizure)
I	Infection (e.g. meningitis)
O	Overdose (too much alcohol or other medicine)
U	Underdose (not taking their medicine with a bad outcome)
T	Trauma
I	Insulin (diabetes with a low blood sugar)
P	Psychological disorder
S	Stroke

Secondary Survey: Characterizing the Pain

C	Character: "What does the pain feel like?"
O	Onset: "When did the pain start?"
L	Location: "Where is the pain located?" Have the victim point with one finger.
D	Duration: "How long does the pain last?"
E	Exacerbation: "What makes the pain worse?"
R	Relief: "What makes the pain better?"
R	Radiation: "Does the pain move (radiate) anywhere?"

Physical Exam

- The physical exam during the secondary survey is a more detailed head-to-toe examination where the rescuer should visibly inspect and palpate (touch) the victim from head to toe, including the back.
- Vital signs helpful to the wilderness responder include:
  - Pulse (in beats per minute): a normal pulse is ~60-100bpm. A high pulse can indicate pain, dehydration or significant blood loss.
  - Respirations (in breaths per minute): normal is 12-20 per minute. Rapid breathing can signify a chest injury or low oxygen; slow breathing can signify brain injury in the proper setting.
  - Skin color, temperature and moisture (SCTM) can be used to signify heat or cold injuries along with allergic reactions and shock (poor blood flow to the whole body).
- A general guide for areas to inspect include the following:
  - Blood or fluid draining from the ears or nose suggests a head injury.
  - Look inside the mouth for loose teeth or other debris that may block the airway.
  - Palpate (push on) the back of the neck (cervical spine) for tenderness and deformities.
  - Palpate (push on) the chest for tenderness (pain when you push on the area).
  - Palpate the abdomen for tenderness (pain when you push on the area).
  - Push on the pelvis from the sides for tenderness or abnormal movement.
  - Examine all four limbs for deformities, tenderness, pulses and if the victim is conscious check, strength and sensation.
- When an abnormality is found, ask the patient if this is an old or new problem.
- Be carefully when checking an area that you think might be injured. Causing pain may make it more difficult to assess the patient thoroughly for the rest of the exam. You should check obvious areas of injury last in order to make it easier to find everything that is wrong.

- When examining an area the patient identifies as painful, start by assessing above and below the injury in order to determine the extent of the injury, before touching the focus of the pain.
- Be aware of "distracting injuries". These are injuries that cause the victim so much pain that they does not notice that they have other injuries. Determining a detailed MOI can help you to anticipate other injuries.
- Examine the patient's back when it is convenient (e.g. when log-rolling the patient) to minimize movement.
- Remember that with an alert and oriented patient, portions of the exam can be replaced by a reliable story of the events leading up to the injury. For example, "I rolled my ankle, didn't fall, and just sat down here on this rock." Such a patient may only require a focused physical exam instead of a complete head-to-toe exam.

Potential Sources of Major Bleeding

- These are potential areas of internal bleeding that are not obvious when just looking at the patient. These are all areas to consider when evaluating a trauma victim and are picked up mostly on the physical examination portion of the secondary survey.
- We use the **CARTS** mnemonic to help remember these potential areas for significant bleeding.

CHEST	The chest is a common source of bleeding, particularly in high-energy trauma. Look for shortness of breath, pain with breathing, and coughing up blood. Examine for chest tenderness, crepitance over the ribs and sternum, flail chest and crackling noises of the chest consistent with air under the skin.
ABDOMEN/PELVIS	Assume abdominal and/or pelvis bleeding in every trauma victim until proven otherwise. Look for bruising over the abdomen and pelvis. Palpate for abdominal and pelvic tenderness on compression.
RENAL	Usually the bleeding is from the kidneys. Look for blood in the urine if you have a prolonged time with the victim. Examine for tenderness of the spine and chest and the lowest level of the ribs.
THIGH	This may occur if there is a femur fracture. Look for deformity, swelling and bruising of the thigh. Palpate for tenderness and crepitance of the thigh.
SKIN/STREET	This is the most obvious place for a rescuer to detect blood. A common error in the wilderness setting is the failure to remove clothing or to roll the patient to look for bleeding. Also, ensure that you survey the area immediately surrounding the victim for a large amount of blood on the ground that may have come from the victim. Specifically, an arterial injury that bleeds significantly may be in spasm at the time you are evaluating the victim and not be an obvious source of bleeding.

Problem List and Plan - SOAP Note

It is essential that at this point you formulate your thoughts as to what the patient's problems are and how you are going to treat them. There may be many problems or there may be only one. Making a problem list and creating a plan is accomplished using a **SOAP** note. This is a systematic note that can assist you in creating an assessment and a treatment plan in a backcountry medical emergency.

Subjective: This is information about the patient – often in the patient's own words. "I have been out in the wind for three hours and I am feeling really cold." You can also include items like age, name, and male or female, adult or child.

Objective: This is information that you gain with your own observations. This is where you will put the SAMPLE history.

Assessment: This is the section where you begin to make a list of what is wrong with the patient.

Plan: For each problem you will write what you are going to do about it.

Remember that if the patient is in critical condition, much of this planning is done in your head rather than writing it down. For example, if someone is not breathing, you would not waste time to write a SOAP note. Instead, you would start CPR.

Ongoing Survey

A unique aspect of wilderness life support is that the rescuer may care for a victim for several hours to days. For this reason, it is important to continue the patient assessment over a longer period of time. The ongoing survey very much depends on the patient's condition, and as such, changes often.
- Initial vitals obtained during the secondary survey should be compared to vitals taken throughout the evacuation or management period. Changes in vitals help alert the rescuer to an improving or deteriorating patient.
- As changes occur, such as the patient's condition, level of responsiveness or the environment, go back to the beginning of the patient assessment.
- If the rescuer has the time and appropriate materials, he or she should try to document the important parts of their evaluation so that this can be handed off to medical professionals later so they have a better understanding of the victim's history.

Spinal Injury Assessment

When evaluating any patient who you know or think has had a traumatic accident, there are a number of steps that need to be taken immediately. In addition to scene safety, assessing for major bleeding and airway management, you must protect the neck or "cervical spine" ("C-spine" for short). This is performed by holding the patient's head on each side and holding it steady to make sure the victim does not move the neck. This is called "holding C-spine". If the C-spine is injured, any motion of the neck caused by the rescuer or the patient may cause injury to the spinal cord. Once you begin holding C-spine, it is extremely important that you do not let go until one of three things happen: 1) you hand-off the patient to a rescuer or professional with a higher level of training, 2) you place the patient on a backboard with head restraints or 3) you determine the likelihood of a C-spine injury is very low. The final option is called "clearing" a C-spine. Ideally a doctor in the hospital does this after transport, however, if holding C-spine will significantly complicate an evacuation and professional evacuation is not an option, it's important to know the steps of clearing a C-spine.

The cervical spine may be cleared and immobilization removed from the patient, if the following clinical preconditions are met.

- The patient must be fully alert and orientated. The patient must not have used alcohol or drugs.
- There must be no tenderness (pain) over the midline (spine) of the back of the neck on direct palpation.

- There must be no neurological issues such as numbness, tingling or weakness in an arm, leg or any part of the body and the patient has not lost control of their bladder or bowel.
- There can be no other injury that is so painful that it may prevent the patient from feeling neck pain. This is called a "distracting" injury.
- A mnemonic that will help the rescuer to remember these criteria is **C-SPINE**. The patient should have NONE of the following.

Spinal Injury Assessment: Clearing a C-spine

C	Cervical midline tenderness
S	Sensory-motor deficit (numbness/weakness)
P	Pain that is bad enough to distract from neck pain
I	Intoxication from alcohol or other drugs
N	Neurological deficit (loss of alertness)
E	Events (sufficient mechanism to cause neck injury)

What constitutes 'sufficient mechanism' is not well defined, but someone who falls from a cliff is more likely to have a neck injury then someone who is walking and then twists his or her ankle.

Provided these criteria are met, the neck may then be examined. If there is no bruising or deformity, no tenderness and a pain free range of active motion, the cervical spine can be "cleared". Determining if there is an unstable C-spine injury and managing it can be difficult, and a missed spine injury can have devastating long-term consequences. So, one must be very cautious in this analysis. Finally, while it is tempting to focus on the cervical spine, it is important to assess and clear the entire spinal column as well. It is also important to remember that commercial neck stabilizing collars or those improvised from SAM splints or clothing are only to serve as a reminder to the patient not to move their neck, they do not actually provide complete neck (spinal) stabilization.

Questions

1. What is the purpose of the blood sweep during the primary survey?
    a. To clear the scene of blood by sweeping it away with a broom
    b. To determine if the victim needs a blood transfusion
    c. To identify sites of major bleeding
    d. To search for internal bleeding

2. You are rock climbing with several of your friends when there is a rock slide and three of your friends fall 10 to 20 feet to the bottom of the cliff. There are also two other people who were injured by falling debris soon afterwards while standing at the bottom of the cliff and looking up. Which one of the following is correct in terms of managing this situation?
    a. You should attempt to move all of the injured people away from the base of the cliff
    b. You should not move anybody as there is a risk of spinal injury by moving them
    c. You should put an overhead shade over those at the base of the cliff but not move them
    d. You should only move those without concern of spinal injury from the base of the cliff

3. A hiker falls down a steep embankment 150 feet and lands at the bottom. She is pale but awake. She has a rapid heart rate of 130 beats / minute and complains of feeling very thirsty. Which one of the following best explains her increased heart rate, paleness and weak pulse?
    a. Deformity of her left wrist without any significant swelling
    b. Deformity, pain, and swelling in her right ankle
    c. Scrapes on her lower legs and hands that are dirty but have no active bleeding
    d. Severe tenderness on palpation of her abdomen

4. Which one of the following is NOT correct in regards to obtaining a history from a patient in the secondary survey?
    a. S = Signs and Symptoms
    b. A = Allergies
    c. M = Medications
    d. P = Past medical history
    e. L = Last meal
    f. E = Exposure to elements

5. Which one of the following is NOT an area that is concerning for internal blood loss in the trauma victim?
    a. Abdomen
    b. Buttocks
    c. Chest
    d. Thigh

6. You are snowshoeing in the mountains during winter. It has been below freezing (32°F / 0°C) most of the day. You come upon a 35-year-old man off to the side of the trail. He is breathing and has a strong regular pulse but is very confused and slow to respond to you. He does not complain of anything. Which one of the following is a potential explanation for his altered mental status?
    a. Intoxication with alcohol
    b. Low blood sugar from too much insulin
    c. Stroke
    d. All of the above should be considered

7. You arrive at the scene of a drowning event. The victim has been pulled from the water and is lying on his back. On your initial assessment the victim is completely unresponsive without any sign of life. Which one of the following is the most appropriate next step in the management of the victim?
    a. Initiate CPR with chest compressions only
    b. Initiate CPR including rescue breaths
    c. Perform a blood sweep
    d. Start rewarming the patient using blankets and body heat

8. Which one of the following is not correct for the Primary Assessment?
    a. M – Massive Hemorrhage
    b. A – Airway with cervical spine stabilization
    c. R – Respiration
    d. C – Crepitation
    e. H – Hypo/Hyperthermia or Hike vs Helicopter

ANSWERS
1. c 2. a 3. d 4. f 5. b 6. d 7. b 8. d

CHAPTER 2

Vital Sign Assessment

Objectives:
- Learn the significance of vital signs and what they measure
- Practice obtaining vital signs from a conscious and unconscious patient

Case 2.1

On a rock-climbing trip, you and a friend, who is a physician, come across a man who has fallen from a steep precipice. You check to verify that the scene is safe and immediately assist the physician in the primary assessment.

Primary Assessment:

Massive Hemorrhage: The patient is bleeding form a large laceration (cut) on the top of his head. There is no other bleeding.

Airway & C-spine: The airway seems to be open. Your friend instructs you to keep the airway open using the jaw-thrust technique and to stabilize the patient's cervical spine.

Respiration: The patient is taking slow shallow breaths. The patient is breathing shallowly.

Circulation: Your friend detects a radial pulse.

Hyper/Hypothermia; Hike vs Helicopter: It is warm and sunny and you are one mile from the trailhead.

- The physician begins a secondary survey by checking the patient's heart rate, respiration rate and skin signs. What do these vital signs tell him?

Vital Signs

What are vital signs?
- The word "vital" refers to items that are essential for life.
- Vital signs are the measurements of these items.
- They are essential to measure early in the assessment of a patient and include the following:
    - Level of consciousness / level of responsiveness (LOC / LOR)
    - Heart rate (HR) or pulse
    - Respiration rate (RR)
    - Skin color, temperature and moisture (SCTM)
    - Body core temperature (T)

Taking and recording vital signs?
- Take (and record) a patient's vital signs as part of the physical exam.
- Consecutive sets of vital signs will help to tell you how the patient is doing.
- Have the same rescuer take the vital signs to help prevent variability.
- In the wilderness, the second set of vitals is often more important than the first, the third set is more important than the second, etc. This is a good way to follow how a patient is progressing.
- Make sure you document the time each set of vital signs was taken.

Level of Consciousness / Responsiveness
- Measure of the brain's ability to relate to the outside world
- Often the FIRST vital sign to noticeably change
- Can be the most difficult to assess accurately

Measurement of LOC
- A - Alert
- V - Verbal
- P - Pain
- U - Unresponsive

Alert
- The patient is awake and able to answer questions appropriately.
- The patient is "oriented" to who they are and some basic situational information
- Each question they answer correctly = oriented by X / 4
    - What's your name?
    - Where are you?
    - What day is it?
    - What happened?
- If they answer all 4 correctly they are oriented by 4 / 4 but if they only know their name, then they are oriented by 1 / 4.

Verbal
- The patient is not alert but does respond in some way when spoken to.
    - Grimacing
    - Grunting
    - Rolling away from rescuer
- The patient may be able to follow simple commands.

Pain
- The patient does not react to talking to him / her but does react to painful stimuli.
- Appropriate responses to pain (such as rubbing their chest vigorously):
    - Pulling away from the rescuer or pushing the rescuer away
    - Groaning or moaning

Unresponsive
- Patient does not respond to any stimuli, to include verbal and painful stimulation.

Heart Rate / Pulse

- The heart rate can be taken anywhere you can palpate a pulse (a pressure wave created by the beating of the heart).
- The radial pulse at the wrist is usually the easiest to check.
- Heart function can be assessed by checking the heart rate, the heart rhythm, and the quality of each heartbeat.
- Rate = number of beats per minute (bpm)
    - Normal = 60-100 bpm in adults. Children typically have a higher heart rate with newborns ranging from 100-150 bpm.
    - Count pulse for 15 seconds and then multiply by four.
- Quality = Force the heart exerts with each beat
    - Normal – a strong easily palpated pulse
    - Thready – weak, indicates inadequate circulation

Respiratory Rate

- Rate = number of breaths/minute
    - Breathing in AND out counts as one breath.
    - Normal = 12-20
    - Count the number of breaths for 30 seconds and multiply by two.
    - Measure the respiratory rate WITHOUT the patient knowing. An easy way to accomplish this is to pretend like you are taking the patient's pulse while secretly counting the respirations.
- Quality
    - Normal = quiet/effortless/easy/unlabored
    - Abnormal = suggests that something may be wrong
        - Too shallow or unusually deep
        - Pained
        - Noisy breathing

Skin Color, Temperature, Moisture

Color
- Look at the color of the patient's skin in non-pigmented areas (lining of eyes, inside of mouth, and fingernail beds). Pink skin is the normal color in these non-pigmented areas.
- Red or flushed skin
    - This happens when the body sends more blood to the skin by widening blood vessels.
    - It may indicate fever or hyperthermia (high body temperature)
- White or pale skin
    - This happens when the body reduces how much blood is being sent to the skin.
    - This often happens when the blood volume is low and hypothermia (low body temperature)
- Blue skin (often called *cyanosis*)
    - Indicates a lack of oxygen in blood

Temperature
- Check skin temperature with the back of your hand.
- Check skin INSIDE of clothing, not on exposed face or hands

Moisture
- Normal skin is slightly moist but feels relatively dry
- Cool and moist skin may indicate poor blood flow due to blood loss or severe dehydration
- Hot and dry skin may indicate unusually high body temperature (hyperthermia)

Body Core Temperature

- Most providers do not carry thermometers with them in the wilderness
- Thermometers that are not always accurate in wilderness:
    - Glass thermometers can be damaged by extreme heat or cold.
    - Standard thermometers do not register hypothermia (low)-range temperatures.
    - Axial (armpit) temperatures are notoriously unreliable.
- Normal – 98.6 °F (37 °C)
- Oral temperature
    - Easy access and accurate
    - Minimal discomfort

Recording Vital Signs

Here is an example of what you might record if you took vitals on a young, healthy person with normal vitals.
- LOC = Alert and oriented to person, place, time and events (A+O×4)
- HR = 70 bpm, regular, strong
- RR = 15 breaths per minute, regular, unlabored
- SCTM = pink, warm, dry

Questions

1. Which of the following changes in vital signs is most consistent with a serious, life-threatening condition?
   a. A change in heart rate of 8 beats per minute
   b. A change in the patient's level of alertness from awake and oriented x 4 to awake and oriented x 1 (name only)
   c. A respiration rate that changes from 16 to 20 over the course of four hours
   d. Skin that changes color six hours after falling 10 feet

2. Which of the following vital signs will change quickly if the patient is in trouble?
   a. Body temperature
   b. Level of consciousness
   c. Skin moisture
   d. All of the above

3. You are measuring the level of consciousness of a victim who fell 10 feet off a cliff. They are not awake, but will respond to you when you talk loudly and ask them to roll over. Where would they fall on the grading scale?
   a. Alert
   b. Verbal
   c. Pain
   d. Unresponsive

ANSWERS
1. b 2. b 3. b

CHAPTER 3
Airway and Breathing

Objectives:
- Understand the importance of an open airway and how it can become obstructed in trauma situations
- Learn how to open and maintain an airway in adults and children
- Learn how to remove a foreign object obstructing a patient's airway
- Review rescue breathing techniques in adults and children

Case 3.1

While you are sitting around a campfire enjoying a freshly roasted marshmallow, two people come frantically running into your campsite. They say that when they were climbing up a rocky ledge 20 yards away from your campsite, a rock came loose and struck their friend. You quickly run to the scene and begin your primary assessment. You immediately notice the girl is not breathing.

- What should you do in this case?
- What are some ways you can open her airway?
- What other precautions should you take while trying to open this girl's airway?

After clearing the scene for safety, prepare to approach the patient and open her airway.
- Gently tap the patient and ask if she is okay.
  - Avoid shaking the victim since her spine has not been cleared of injury.
  - Place the patient on their back.
  - Do this by rolling the person while stabilizing the neck.

The Airway

An open airway signifies that air is able to flow freely from the mouth or nose to the lungs. The tongue often blocks the airway in cases where the patient is unconscious and laying on their back. The unconscious victim does not "swallow their tongue". Instead, the tongue is attached to the mouth but will relax backwards and may block full flow of air down into the lungs.

One of two maneuvers can be used to open the airway:
- Head-Tilt/Chin-Lift Maneuver
- Jaw-Thrust Maneuver

Head-Tilt/Chin-Lift Maneuver

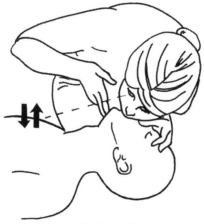

Figure 3.1 Head-Tilt/Chin Maneuver

1. Tilt the head back by placing pressure on the forehead and lift the chin as shown.
2. When lifting the chin, apply upward pressure on the bone (avoid pressing on the soft tissue below as this may further block the airway).
3. Continue until chin points to sky. In children, place head in neutral position.

Jaw-Thrust Maneuver

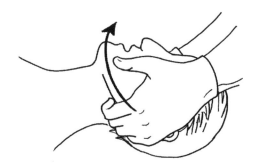

Figure 3.2 Jaw-Thrust Maneuver

1. Kneel at the victim's head facing the victim's feet.
2. Put arms in such a position that creates a continuous line with the patient's spine.
3. Place thumbs on cheekbones and two or three fingers at the corner of the patient's jaw (at the angle between chin and ear).
4. Use counter pressure from your thumbs on the patient's cheekbones to pull the jaw forward with your fingers.
    - Assess the patient's breathing.
    - A breathless patient requires foreign-body removal and/or rescue breathing.

Foreign-Body Airway Obstruction: Conscious Adult and Child (Heimlich Maneuver)

1. Wrap arms around the person's waist from behind (keep elbows out from ribs).
2. Make a fist and place thumb in on midline abdomen above navel and well below the bottom of the sternum (breastbone).
3. Grab your fist with your second hand and pull quickly in and up in a powerful motion.
4. Repeat until airway clears or until the patient goes unconscious.

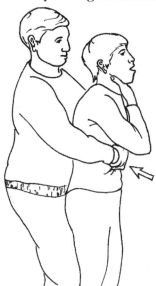

Figure 3.3 Heimlich Maneuver.

Foreign-Body Airway Obstruction: Unconscious Adult

1. The victim should be lowered to the ground and CPR should be initiated.

Foreign-Body Airway Obstruction: Conscious Infant Less than One Year Old

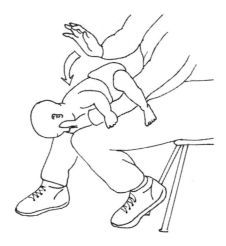

Figure 3.4 Foreign-Body Airway Obstrution in Conscious Infant less than 1 Year Old

1. Determine why there is a lack of breath
2. Hold infant as shown in the image above, supporting the head with the head positioned lower than the trunk.
3. Give five forceful blows between shoulder blades with the heel of your hand.
4. Using the hand that was used to give the blows, support the neck and back of the baby's head while turning the baby on its back, then give five chest thrusts with the finger of your free hand on the lower half of the baby's sternum.
5. Repeat until the breathing is clear or until the baby is unconscious.

Foreign-Body Airway Obstruction: Unconscious Infant Less than One Year Old

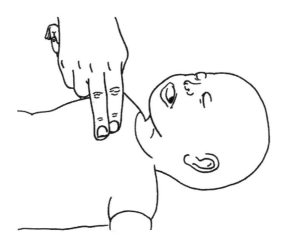

Figure 3.5 Foreign-Body Airway Obstruction in Unconscious Infant less than 1 year old

1. Open the airway using tongue-jaw lift maneuver. Look for obstruction—**DO NOT** blind finger sweep.
2. Open the airway and ventilate by sealing your mouth over the patient's mouth **and nose** and breathe out slowly so the baby's chest rises.
3. If the first attempt fails, reposition the airway and try a second time.
4. If the airway is still blocked, give five back blows then five chest thrusts.
5. Repeat steps 1-3 until the airway is opened.
6. If the baby is still not breathing once the airway is open, start CPR.

Rescue Breathing Review

1. In most situations, hands only CPR should be performed without any rescue breathing.
2. Those unique wilderness situations that may require rescue breathing as part of CPR include drowning, lightning strike and avalanche burial.
3. If you are going to perform rescue breathing on a victim, you should use barrier protection to keep yourself safe. This is especially true in light of the fact that rescue breathing is only really indicated in drowning, lightning and avalanche burial.
4. Start all sessions with 30 chest compressions before initiating the rescue breathing.
5. Pinch the patient's nostrils and hold the mouth open.
6. Take a deep breath away from the patient's mouth.
7. Seal your mouth over the patient's mouth.
8. Give two breaths over one second each making sure to see the chest rise for each one.
9. If you cannot see the chest rising, reposition the airway and try again.
10. Check for pulse: If it is present, continue breathing. If there is no pulse, start CPR.
11. Use one breath per five seconds.
12. Rescue breathing can be done mouth to mouth or mouth to nose if necessary.

Rescue Breathing Exceptions in Children and Infants

1. Do not tilt the child's head too far back as this may actually block the airway in young patients.
2. If you are going to perform rescue breathing on a victim, you should use barrier protection to keep yourself safe.
2. Seal off mouth and nose with your mouth.
3. Use small puffs instead of full breaths.
4. Watch the patient's chest and abdomen.
5. Use one breath per three seconds.

Questions

1. **When preparing to open an airway, what is the first thing you should do?**
   a. Give the person a painful stimulus to their chest to see if they respond
   b. Move the person to a sitting position, then rotate their head from side to side to see if any objects protrude from their throat
   c. Roll the person onto his or her side and press their chin into their chest
   d. Tap on the person and ask if they are okay

2. **An adult has a foreign body obstructing their airway and you decide to perform the Heimlich maneuver. Which one of the following is NOT a step?**
   a. Place the thumb of one hand on the middle of the patient's abdomen above the navel
   b. Repeat thrusts until the airway clears or the patient goes unconscious
   c. With your second hand, grasp throat and check for position of foreign object
   d. With your second hand on your first hand, press in and upward with powerful motion

3. **Which of the following maneuvers do you use to open the airway of a person whom you suspect has a spine injury?**
   a. Head-Tilt/Chin-Lift Maneuver
   b. Jaw-Thrust Maneuver
   c. Tongue-Jaw Lift Maneuver

4. **In a conscious infant who is six months old, which one of the following is appropriate in removing a foreign body from the airway?**
   a. Blind finger sweep
   b. Give five forceful blows between shoulder blades with heel of hand
   c. Give the infant five abdominal thrusts in the mid abdomen
   d. Hold the infant by the feet and shake the body in an up and down motion

ANSWERS
1. d 2. c 3. b 4. b

CHAPTER 4
Bleeding and Shock

Objectives:
- Understand the dangers of bleeding and demonstrate how to control bleeding using various techniques
- Be able to describe specific causes, stages, and symptoms of shock
- Be able to demonstrate how to manage a patient in shock

Case 4.1

You are mountain biking outside Yosemite National Park when one of your friends falls violently on a rocky downhill section of trail. As he stands back up to dust himself off, you notice a lot of blood running from his right thigh. He has landed on a sharp rock in the trail that has cut deeply into his inner thigh. Bright red blood is pouring from the laceration.

- What would you do?
- Do you need to stop his bleeding or will it stop on its own?
- What steps will you take to control the bleeding?
- An understanding of bleeding and how to control life-threatening bleeding is a critical technique that you must learn

The Heart

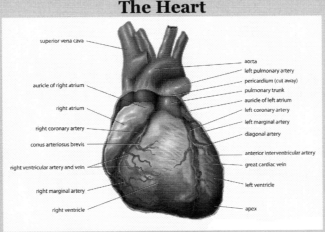

Figure 4.1 The Human Heart

- The heart is a large muscle that pumps blood to the whole body.
- Tracking Blood Flow
    - (From large to small): heart – arteries – capillaries – veins (and then back to the heart)

Hemorrhage: Bleeding From A Wound

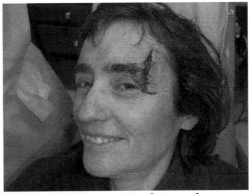

Figure 4.2 Head Wound

- Bleeding (*hemorrhage*) can occur inside the body (internal) or involving the outside of the body (external). Hemorrhage can be classified by the type of vessel that has been injured. The following list helps to identify what type of vessel has been injured:
    o Capillary bleeding – slow oozing and bright red in color
    o Venous bleeding – steady flow and dark maroon (due to lower oxygen in the veins)
    o Arterial bleeding – under high pressure, often spurting and brighter red in color

- Most capillary and small venous hemorrhaging will stop bleeding without your assistance. However, larger wounds and arterial damage will usually require your assistance to stop the bleeding.

Control of External Bleeding

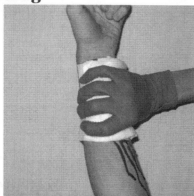

Figure 4.3 Pressure to Control External Bleeding

First Step: Direct Pressure

- The first method is to apply direct pressure on the wound
- When applying direct pressure, remember to follow these rules:
    o Use gloves and sterile dressing (if available) to reduce the chance of infection
    o Apply pressure with the heel of hand directly onto wound for 10-20 minutes
    o Raise the wound above the level of the heart, if possible
    o Be patient
- Certain wounds are more difficult to control the bleeding
    o Large wounds: because of the large number of blood vessels involved and it is harder to put pressure on the entire wound
    o Scalp wounds: because the scalp has a lot of blood vessels

Second Step: Pressure Dressing +/- Hemostatic Dressing

- A pressure bandage should be applied if there is continued bleeding or if you need your hands to provide other care to the patient.
- How to apply a pressure dressing:
    o Wrap and hold the dressing in place with an elastic bandage (Ace® wrap) or tape that is wrapped circumferentially around the extremity.
    o If you have a special "hemostatic" dressing which is specifically designed to stop bleeding then you should apply this directly to the wound and then wrap it with a pressure dressing.
    o If the patient continues to bleed through the pressure dressing, then you should remove the elastic bandage and place additional dressing on top of the dressing that is already on the wound.
        ➢ Do not remove that initial dressing
        ➢ Wrap this additional dressing with elastic bandage
        ➢ Apply direct pressure with your hand on top of this pressure dressing
    o After applying a pressure bandage, be sure to check distal function and pulse often

Third Step: Using a Tourniquet

- While widely viewed as a last resort, a tourniquet can be used initially for a short interval of time to determine the best approach of treatment and evacuation. If you decide to use a tourniquet in this fashion, do not leave it for more than five minutes.
- If you have tried the other methods to stop the bleeding and the wound in continuing to bleed a lot through the dressing, then you should consider a tourniquet as a last resort, if you are able to place one.
- For full directions on tourniquet placement, see the Wound chapter.
- Always note the time the tourniquet was applied. Writing the time on the victim's forehead is very effective because it is obvious to other rescuers and to the providers who receive the victim as they are brought into a hospital setting.

Internal Bleeding

- Bleeding into a body cavity is life-threatening.
- Patients can bleed internally anywhere, but there are specific areas of the body (CARTS) that more easily allow for life threatening bleeding:
    - Chest
    - Abdomen / Pelvis (usually due to a spleen and/or liver injury or pelvis fracture)
    - Renal/Retroperitoneal (kidney area in the back)
    - Thigh (From a broken femur / thigh bone)
    - Skin / Street (External bleeding that was significant and then slowed down)
- Patient may lose a lot of blood before you are aware of any bleeding because it is not obvious to you
- Carefully assess injuries to CARTS
    - Look for external bruising, guarding, and an increasingly abdominal pain.
    - There is little treatment that can be done while in the field for internal bleeding
    - Stabilize injuries
    - Keep the patient warm
- Initiate rapid evacuation if you have any concern of internal bleeding

Shock

Shock is defined as the lack of blood flow to vital organs, including the brain

Causes of Shock

- All shock results from failure of one or more of the components of the cardiovascular system.
- Cardiogenic Shock
    - Failure of the heart
    - Heart attack – muscle damage due to lack of blood supply
    - Trauma to heart

- Hypovolemic Shock
    - Caused by a low fluid volume
    - This occurs with severe bleeding, dehydration and burns

- Vasogenic Shock
    - Caused by low resistance to blood flow within the blood vessels
    - This means that the vessels enlarge (dilate) and the heart cannot maintain blood flow.
    - Occurs with severe allergies (anaphylaxis), spinal injuries and infection

Symptoms of Shock

- These stages are not important to memorize. Rather, it is the progression and the signs and symptoms of shock that are important to recognize.
- Stage 1: Compensatory Shock
  - Anxiety, confusion, restlessness, pale and cool skin
  - Increased pulse and respiration rate
  - Patients showing these declines in vital signs should be <u>evacuated</u>.

- Stage 2: Decompensated Shock
  - Altered level of consciousness, cold and clammy skin
  - Rapid weak pulse and respirations
  - It may be hard to find a pulse

- Stage 3: Irreversible Shock
  - Drowsy, unresponsive, cold skin
  - Slow heart rate and slow, labored respirations
  - No pulses palpable

Special Risk Factors of Shock

- <u>Children and teenagers</u> – At these ages, it can be hard to tell that they are in shock as their bodies tend to be more resilient and compensate for a longer period of time against signs of shock, essentially masking the severity of the condition.
- <u>Elderly</u> – Elderly are the opposite of children and young adolescents, as their bodies do not compensate as well and have an even earlier onset of shock.

Management of Shock

Anticipate and treat for shock until you have ruled it out.

1. Early intervention is very important
2. Treat the underlying cause (when possible)
3. Stop bleeding, splint fractures
4. Insulate from cold or protect from heat
5. Monitor vital signs frequently
6. Patients with a good level of consciousness should drink to keep hydrated
7. Evacuate as soon as possible

Evacuation Guidelines

Initiate rapid evacuation for all patients suspected of going into shock.

Review

1. Direct pressure and elevation to stop or slow bleeding
2. Remember to check for internal bleeding (CARTS)
3. Shock occurs when there is a lack of blood to vital organs
4. Management of shock
   - Be looking for it
   - Treat causes if you can recognize them
   - Maintain body temperature
   - Monitor vitals
   - Orally rehydrate if the patient is alert enough to drink
   - Evacuate at the first concern of shock

Questions

1. **Which of the following describes venous bleeding?**
    a. Bubbling and very thin
    b. High pressure, often spurting and brighter red
    c. Slow oozing and bright red
    d. Steady flow and dark maroon

2. **Which one of the following is correct regarding the management of a victim of hemorrhagic (bleeding) shock in the wilderness?**
    a. Cooling the patient down with ice, even if they are cold
    b. Delay evacuation until you find the source of the bleeding
    c. Giving liquids if the patient is alert enough to drink
    d. Treating the patient with alcohol to help treat the pain

3. **Which of the following is NOT a body cavity usually associated with being able to bleed to death into?**
    a. Chest
    b. Forearm
    c. Renal/retroperitoneal
    d. Thigh

ANSWERS
1. d 2. c 3. b

CHAPTER 5
Abdominal and Chest Injuries

Objectives:
- Describe the basic anatomy of the abdomen and chest
- Describe the general signs and symptoms of abdominal and chest injuries
- Describe the general treatment for abdominal and chest injuries
- Demonstrate specific treatment for blunt and penetrating abdominal trauma
- Demonstrate specific treatment for chest trauma

Abdominal Trauma

Case 5.1

You are camping in the mountains when you hear a friend scream. When you get to her, you notice that she has fallen off of a large rock, landing on a small boulder. She is complaining of abdominal pain and holding her abdomen.

The abdomen is commonly separated into four areas called "quadrants" that are used to help diagnose the origin of the abdominal pain and locate internal organs.

Right upper quadrant (RUQ)
Right lower quadrant (RLQ)

Left upper quadrant (LUQ)
Left lower quadrant (LLQ)

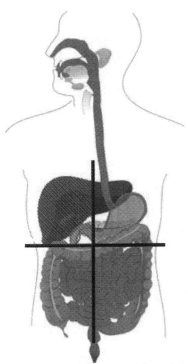
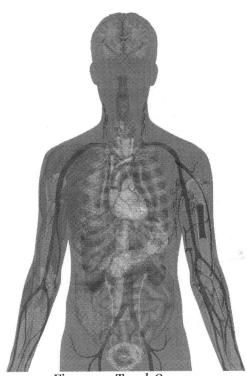

Figure 5.1 Four Quadrants of the Abdomen   *Figure 5.2 Trunk Organs*

The RUQ contains:
- Liver, right kidney (lies closer to the back than the abdomen) and gall bladder

The LUQ contains:
- Spleen, stomach, and left kidney (lies closer to the back than the abdomen)

The RLQ contains:
- Small intestine including the appendix and the large intestine
- In females the right lower quadrant also contains the right ovary

The LLQ contains:
- Small intestine and the large intestine
- In females the left lower quadrant also contains the left ovary

Steps of an Abdominal Assessment

- Determine the mechanism of injury (MOI)
- Upon knowing the mechanism of injury, determine what kind of damage could have been done
- Does the mechanism of injury indicate possible injury to the abdomen or merit concern?
- Is the patient moving or staying still?
- Does the patient appear to be in a great deal of pain?
- Look at the patient's abdomen while they are lying down
- Look for symmetry as well as normal shaping of the abdomen
- Look for signs of trauma such as the following:
    - Penetrating wounds
    - Bruising
- Feel the abdomen by gently applying pressure in each of the four quadrants
- Look for pain, tenderness, firmness and rigid muscles
- Monitor vital signs. If there is internal bleeding, the patient could go into shock.
- Ask the patient if they have had blood in their urine, stool, or vomit as this can indicate internal bleeding.

Trauma

There are two types of trauma that need to be evaluated in an abdominal assessment:
1. Blunt trauma
2. Penetrating trauma

Blunt trauma
- Usually occurs from a forceful blow to the abdomen. First determine the mechanism of injury and events leading up to the injury. Ask the patient and/ or bystanders to give you a description of the accident as this can give you an idea of what injury the patient could have sustained. Always assume the worst-case scenario before clearing an injury.

- Performing a general abdominal assessment:
    - Be especially aware of bruising as it is a sign of potentially significant injury
    - Be aware of the abdomen becoming more firm (due to internal bleeding).
    - See if the patient "guards" against pressure in any quadrant during the assessment. Guarding is when the patient has pain and does not want you to push on that area.
    - Be aware of peritonitis

    *Peritonitis is an inflammatory reaction within the abdomen due to bleeding, infection or significant injury to the vital organs. It is described as a sharp, stabbing, or burning pain. The patient will be in a considerable amount of pain, so much that they will not want to move. In order to alleviate the pain by decreasing pressure on the abdomen, the patient may assume the fetal position.

- Signs and symptoms of abdominal injuries
    - Nausea and vomiting
    - Blood in the patient's urine, stool or vomit
    - Increased respirations and elevated heart rate
    - Fever may develop, especially if patient develops peritonitis

- Treatment of abdominal injuries
    - Follow the MARCH guidelines
    - Keep patient still and warm
    - Avoid giving the patient anything to eat or drink
    - If it is a long evacuation, patient may have small sips of a cool liquid
    - Do not give the patient alcohol

Penetrating Trauma
- Occurs when an object passes through or penetrates into the abdomen.
- Bleeding can be rapid and lethal. If your patient is in shock or going into shock, their only chance of survival depends on immediate evacuation.
- If patient is stable and does not go into shock, infection is a bigger concern.
- Assessment: Same as for a blunt trauma.
- Treatment:
  - Generally the same supportive care as you do for blunt trauma
  - Specific treatment depends on the degree of soft tissue injury
  - Control bleeding
  - Clean all wounds
  - Do NOT remove an impaled object.
    - The reason you do not remove the object is that it may cause more damage on its way out as well stopping some bleeding that will break free when it is removed.
    - Instead, place padding around the object so that it does not penetrate further or get accidently pulled out.
  - Evacuate the patient as soon as possible.

- Evisceration: This is when the intestines protrude out of the injured site
  - Remove all clothing from around the wound
  - Apply a bandage soaked in clean as water over the exposed intestine
  - Apply another layer of dressing to prevent the dressing from drying out
  - Cover with a thick dry dressing
  - Evacuate immediately

Chest Trauma

Case 5.2

A young man falls while hanging food in a tree – he falls, scraping his arms and legs. He quickly develops shallow breathing because it hurts on the side of his chest. You notice blood in that same area and pull back the shirt to see a shallow cut. There is tenderness at a very specific point. He is alert. The bleeding is superficial, and while he has painful breathing it is not getting worse. His chest expands equally on both sides.

Anatomy of the Chest

- Twelve ribs on each side protect the chest
- All the ribs are connected to the spine in the back
- The top 10 ribs are connected in the front to the sternum either directly or by cartilage, while the bottom two 'float' in the chest wall.
- The lungs fill both sides of the chest and the heart is on the left side.
- On the bottom of the chest cavity is a domed muscle that appears like a shelf – called the diaphragm. This is the main muscle that causes humans to breathe. There are other muscles that are in between the ribs, called the intercostal muscles that expand the rib cage and help, usually with heavy breathing.
- When a person takes in a breath, the diaphragm drops down, expanding the chest cavity, causing a decrease in pressure. Air rushes to fill this void. This is called the active phase of breathing. When the diaphragm relaxes, air is pushed back out through in what is called the passive phase of breathing.

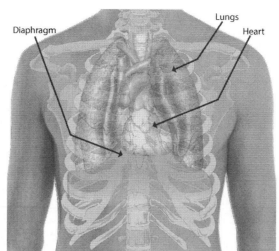
Figure 5.3 Anatomy of the Chest

Common Chest Injuries

Chest injuries are common. Most are not serious, but some are life threatening. When you examine someone for a chest injury there are several important points to remember.

- Examine the chest - Look for blood, bruising or broken skin.
- Look at the rate and depth of breathing – is the patient breathing faster or shallower?
- Look at the ease of breathing - is the patient having more trouble breathing?
- Look at the sputum (saliva) – is there blood in the saliva?

A patient that has point tenderness on the chest wall and is breathing much faster and is also having trouble breathing should make you aware of a more serious situation. If the patient is coughing up blood this would also heighten your concern.

Fractured (broken) or injured rib
- A very common chest injury
- Usually not life threatening
- A fractured rib can puncture a lung (pneumothorax – mentioned below), so watch for this
- These are very painful and there is pain and tenderness at a very specific point over the injury site ("point tenderness")
- The patient's breathing is usually more shallow because of the pain
- Often, there will be bruising at the site of injury.
- Patients with minor fractures need little done
- If the symptoms worsen, consider one of the more serious conditions below

Pneumothorax
- Literally this means "air in the chest"
- This can be very life threatening if air keeps leaking from the injured lung as it can collapse the heart and the blood vessels leading to the heart in addition to the lung.
- Signs and Symptoms:
    - Sharp chest pain
    - Difficulty breathing
    - Anxiety
    - Rapid pulse
    - Bruising
    - Pale, cool, clammy skin (signs of shock)

- Treat similar to rib fracture:
  - Oxygen if available
  - Semi - reclining is usually a better position
  - Immediate evacuation

Sucking chest wound
- Penetration of chest
- Hole in chest wall
- Bubbling sound while breathing
- Air moves in and sometimes out of hole
- Air sucked through the hole collapses the lung
- Signs and Symptoms:
  - Difficulty breathing
  - Moist sucking sound / bubbling of air at the injury site
  - Anxiety
  - Rapid pulse
  - Pale, cool, clammy skin (shock)

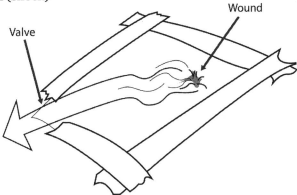

Figure 5.4 Treatment for Sucking Chest Wound

- Treatment:
  - Cover the hole with a glove or piece of plastic
  - Leave one corner free so that air can exit but not enter
  - If air doesn't leave then a larger pneumothorax can develop

Hemothorax
- Broken ribs can tear a vessel and cause blood to collect around the lung in the chest
- Blood can pool around the lung and prevent expansion of lungs
- Breath sounds may diminish
- May see blood in sputum (hemoptysis)
- Signs and Symptoms
  - Sharp chest pain
  - Difficulty breathing
  - Anxiety
  - Rapid pulse
  - Possibility of hemoptysis
  - Pale, cool, clammy skin
- Treatment – same as pneumothorax and immediate evacuation

General Chest Injury Guidelines

- Keep airway open
- Inspect bare chest: look, ask, feel
- Treat any injury
- If possible, let patient get into the position that is most comfortable to them

Questions

1. Which one of the following is found in the right upper quadrant (RUQ) of the abdomen?
    a. Liver
    b. Ovary
    c. Small intestine
    d. Spleen

2. You are biking in Moab when you come across a man who is clutching his abdomen in pain. He said he crashed on his bike half an hour ago and the handle bars were thrust into his abdomen. He has bruising in his right upper quadrant and has significant tenderness in that area when you push on it. What should you do?
    a. Ask the man to try walking and give him some food to eat
    b. Keep the man still and warm as you look for an evacuation route but avoid food and water
    c. Use alcohol to dull the pain
    d. Wrap a tight bandage around his abdomen

3. A person falls landing on his chest. He has immediate pain. Within a few minutes he begins to have extreme shortness of breath and increased chest pain. His most likely diagnosis?
    a. Heart attack
    b. Liver injury
    c. Pneumothorax
    d. Spleen injury

4. While backpacking, you come across a woman who fell from a tree and landed on a branch below, causing a small branch to penetrate her abdomen in the left lower quadrant (LLQ). She seems alert and is having only moderate amounts of pain. When you observe the wound, you are not sure how far it has penetrated but it is bleeding a moderate amount. What is the most worrisome immediate complication that should be addressed?
    a. Bleeding
    b. Infection
    c. Pain
    d. Pneumothorax

ANSWERS
1. a 2. b 3. c 4. a

CHAPTER 6
Musculoskeletal Injuries

Objectives:
- To properly use the medical terms of sprain, dislocation, open fracture and closed fracture
- Be able to properly manage dislocations, strains and sprains
- Recognize signs and symptoms of simple and open fractures
- Understand and demonstrate proper splinting techniques
- Describe when and how you would realign and splint fractures in the wilderness setting
- Identify and treat life-threatening musculoskeletal injuries

Evaluation and Treatment of Musculoskeletal Injuries

Basic Evaluation

- Determine the mechanism of injury
- Examine the area for swelling, discoloration and tenderness over the injury site
- Examine the range of motion of the injured joint, if the patient can tolerate this, it might be possible to use the injured joint
- The most important factor is the patient's ability to use the injury
  - Can the patient complete the wilderness activity?
  - Is the patient able to walk to definitive care?

RICES for Basic Treatment of Musculoskeletal injuries
- RICES is the acronym that is used to help treat injuries
- This helps by treating pain and may help to reduce swelling
- Follow the RICES treatment for the first 72 hours following the injury.
  - **R**est: Rest the injured area from activity and stress. Immobilize it if necessary.
  - **I**ce: Apply ice or cold packs for 15-20 minutes, with at least 30 minutes before reapplying.
  - **C**ompression: A compression wrap may be helpful for some joint injuries. The wrap should compress the joint, but not so tightly that it restricts circulation.
  - **E**levate: Elevate the joint above the level of the victim's heart to help minimize swelling.
  - **S**tabilization: Immobilize the injured joint for transport.

Types of Musculoskeletal Injuries

Sprains

- A sprain involves the ligaments (tissue that connects bone to bone) of a joint and means that the ligaments have been stretched or even torn.
- A sprain usually occurs when a joint is twisted or wrenched beyond the normal range of motion that causes the ligaments to stretch or tear.
- While sprains can occur in any joint in the body they happen most often in the ankles. Symptoms include pain, swelling, and discoloration of the injured joint.
- Sprains can be difficult to differentiate from fractures, due to the fact that they share many of the same signs and symptoms.

Treatment of Sprains
- RICES therapy
- Patient's frequently cannot use the affected joint
- May need help to walk. If this is a knee or ankle – litter evacuation may be needed

Strains

- Strains, unlike a sprain, involve tendons that are the fibrous bands that connect muscles to bones and facilitate the movement of our limbs.
- A strain, simply put, is fatigue due to overuse or strenuous movements.
- While strains are usually considered to be minor injuries, they can cause pain and discomfort.

Treatment of Strains
- RICES therapy
- The best way to deal with strains is to try and minimize the use of the limb that is causing pain.

Tendonitis

- This is the inflammation of a tendon because of overuse.
- This is common in sports where the participant will use a tendon repeatedly, such as in paddling or hiking.
- These symptoms may be minor and annoying or completely limiting.

Treatment of Tendonitis
- The best treatment is to decrease the use of the joint.
- This might be impossible given the circumstances.
- RICES therapy

Dislocations

- A dislocation occurs when a sufficient force (a push or a pull) is placed on a joint that causes a bone to come out of its socket.
- Dislocations are most common in the shoulder, elbow, finger, and kneecap.
- While dislocations themselves can create quite an ordeal, the real damage is usually caused to blood vessels, nerves, muscle and ligaments.
- Signs and symptoms of a dislocation include:
  - Deformity is usually very evident.
  - Severe pain of the joint and with any attempted movement of the joint.
  - Inability to move a joint because of pain.
- Our bodies are symmetrical so comparing a joint to the uninjured side may be helpful in being able to determine if a dislocation has occurred.

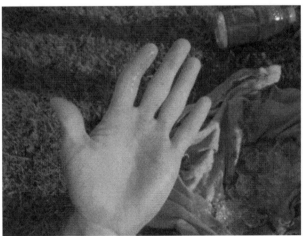

Figure 6.1

Treatment of Dislocations
- After a dislocation occurs the muscles that surround the joint will begin to spasm, making it harder to reduce the dislocated limb.
- This makes putting the joint back into place (reduction) more difficult with time
- If you have not been trained to reduce a joint dislocation, then you should immobilize the injured joint in a comfortable position and initiate evacuation as soon as possible
- If you know how to reduce a dislocated joint, then the sooner after the injury it is attempted the higher the chance that you will be able to reduce.
- Reducing the dislocation will also be helpful in providing pain relief.

Reduction
- You should not attempt to reduce a dislocated joint unless you have been trained, as you may cause more harm if you do it incorrectly.
- These are general directions to reinforce / refresh previous training that you may have had with joint reduction
    - Place yourself comfortably
    - Take a firm grip distal (at the end of the limb) to the injury and provide traction-in-line. This means you should pull from the end of the limb as if you are straightening it out.
    - Pull with a steady and slowly increasing force without jerking.
    - Gently move extremity toward normal alignment, do not use force
    - Stop if pain increases, most patients will feel relocation take place and immediately feel relief

After Reduction
- Splint the joint with plenty of padding
- Ice the joint to minimize swelling
- Check for sensation and circulation distal to the injury
- Most dislocations should be evacuated for definitive medical care
- Dislocations that resist reduction should be evacuated immediately
- Dislocation of fingers or toes and chronic dislocations don't need to be evacuated if joint is usable

Fractures

- A fracture is any break or crack in a bone
- There are two general types of fractures: closed and open
- **Closed fracture**
    - In this case the bone is broken but has not punctured the skin exposing the bone.
    - If a closed fracture is left untreated or handled improperly, it can progress into an open fracture.
    - If you suspect a bone fracture, DO NOT try to move the suspected injury to test for pain.

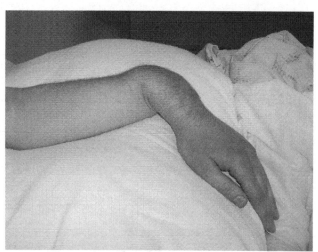

Figure 6.2 Closed fracture "false joint"

- **Open (compound) fracture**
    - Just like a closed fracture the bone is broken except in this case the fractured bone has punctured the skin creating an open wound.
    - Be aware that the bone does not need to be protruding out to be considered an open fracture.
    - This may happen when the broken bone cuts through the skin, or when an object breaks the skin as it fractures the bone.
    - Open fractures cause more concern because the open wound allows bacteria and other foreign debris into the fracture.
    - Such bacteria and debris can ultimately lead to serious bone or other tissue infection.

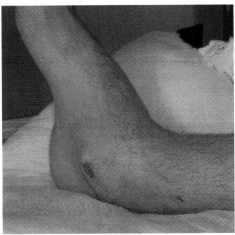
Figure 6.3 Open ankle fracture

- Since fractures can be difficult to diagnose without x-rays the following signs may help to indicate where there is a fracture (Note that even with these guidelines it will not be possible to identify all bone fractures):
  o Point tenderness - pain and tenderness at a very specific point of the body
  o Deformity – as mentioned before our bodies are symmetrical so if there is an abnormal shape position, or motion of a bone/joint then a fracture could be present
  o Inability to use the extremity – a bone fracture can most likely render the limb unusable. If a victim cannot move the limb or joint, or cannot bear weight on it, a fracture should be suspected.
  o Swelling and bruising – at or around the fracture site
  o False joint – the ability to move a limb at a point where no joint formally exists
  o Bone snap – sometimes the victim will hear or feel a bone snap which can help to diagnose a bone fracture
  o Crepitation - the grinding of bones that can sometimes be heard moving a fractured bone

A sprain and a fracture are sometimes difficult to differentiate. If you are not sure which injury the victim has, then splint the extremity and assume it is fractured.

Treatment of Fractures

Since fractures and dislocation injuries are very serious injuries it is important to thoroughly examine them. Here are some general guidelines to help in the process of determining if an individual has suffered a musculoskeletal injury:

- If the mechanism of injury is unknown or such that a neck or back injury is suspected, immobilize the neck immediately upon reaching the victim.
- Completely uncover the injured area to look for deformity, swelling, discoloration, breaks in the skin consistent with an open fracture, and other associated injuries.
- Gently palpate (feel) the injured area for tenderness, abnormal movement, and crepitation.
- Check for numbness or altered sensation beyond the injury.
- Check circulation beyond the injury by pinching the fingernail or toenail bed (if the injury is to an arm or leg) and see how long it takes for the color to return to normal (from white to pink). It should be less than 3 seconds.

Splinting Basics
- The main reason for splinting an injury is to immobilize a limb so as to not worsen an injury and to reduce the pain.
- General principles regarding splinting include:
  o A splint should be long enough to immobilize the joints both above and below the site of injury
  o The splint should immobilize the fractured limb in its functional position
    ➢ The leg should be splinted with a slight bend at the knee

- The ankle and elbow should be splinted with the joints flexed at a 90-degree angle
- The wrist should be splinted slightly bent backwards (extended)
- The fingers should be bent (flexed) in a position similar to that of holding a can of soda and should have loose swath or cloth in between each finger to ensure proper blood as well as lymph flow
  - Remove ALL (including sentimental) jewelry and accessories, such as watches, bracelets, and rings, before applying a splint. Swelling due to injury will make these objects very hard to remove if left in place.
  - Use padding within the splint to make it as comfortable as possible. Use plenty of padding at bony area, such as elbows, knees, and ankles.
  - Splints should be made from rigid, sturdy material. Examples are sticks, boards, skis, paddles, heavy cardboard, and rolled up magazines or newspapers. Be creative when creating trying to conjure materials for a splint. Soft metallic splints are a must for any outdoor first aid kit.
  - Secure the splint in place with pack or lifejacket straps, tape, belts, strips of cloth, webbing, or rope. Tie securely, but not tightly enough to inhibit distal function or blood flow to the limb. Secure the splint in several places, both above and below the fracture, sprain or dislocation. Do not secure a splint directly over the injured area.
  - Avoid moving the injured area unnecessarily
  - Mold the splint on the uninjured limb or body part first and then transfer it to the correct site
  - After splinting, elevate the injured body part to minimize swelling
  - Always recheck sensation and circulation beyond the site of injury after placing a splint. If sensation and circulation is inhibited due to splinting, redo the splint.
  - Frequently check circulation distal to the injury and splint. If circulation is or begins to be inhibited loosen or reposition the splint to allow proper blood flow.

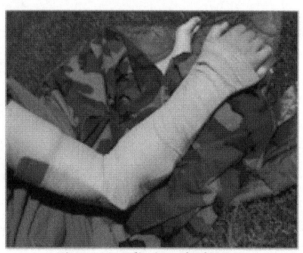

Figure 6.4 Splinting of a forearm

Realignment of a Closed Fracture
It is not necessary to realign a fractured limb unless distal function and circulation is restricted. At your level of training, it would be very unlikely that you would attempt to reduce a fracture that is closed. However, we describe how to do this in the rare event you are in a situation where you must do this to save the limb due to poor circulation.

Realignment of a closed fracture can be accomplished by:
- Straighten the limb by pulling on it below the fracture in a direction that will straighten it. This should be done while someone else holds the limb above the fracture.
- While continuing to hold the limb straight, apply a splint to prevent further motion.
- Check distal function and sensation after realignment often and track the limb's progress.

Realignment of an Open Fracture
Reasons for realigning an open fracture are fundamentally the same as for realigning a closed fracture. The procedure for aligning a closed fracture is similar to an open fracture but also includes the following:

- The wound and extruding parts of the bone should be thoroughly irrigated and removed of all foreign matter. Although risk of infection is present, it may be necessary to replace the exposed bone end back into the wound during traction for proper realignment.
- While continuing to hold the limb straight, apply a splint to prevent further motion.
- Cover the wound with a sterile dressing, then bandage.
- Check and recheck distal function, sensation, and function often after realigning an open fracture.

Pelvic Fractures
- Pelvic fractures call for rapid evacuation due to the risk of significant bleeding.
- Place a sweatshirt or jacket around the pelvis and create a knot that gently secures the fractured pelvis into place.
- In the most comfortable position for the victim create a splint by placing padding between the legs and then by strapping the legs together.
- Do not elevate the legs.
- Refrain from pressing on the pelvis unless absolutely necessary. Each time you press on a pelvic fracture, you will move the bones and may worsen the bleeding.

Femur Fractures
- Fracture of the thigh bone (called the femur) is an important problem to identify since these fractures can cause significant bleeding.
- Splint the injured leg to the good leg by tying them together and recheck sensation and circulation in the foot often.

Prevention

These are some guidelines that will help to prevent musculoskeletal injuries in the backcountry:

- Make sure all footwear fits properly and is in good shape. Ankle and knee injuries are among the most common musculoskeletal injuries reported in the wilderness.
- Ensure backpacks fit properly and are loaded with the heaviest items closest to the back with lighter items loaded toward the outside.
- Always use proper safety gear with secondary safety systems when participating in dangerous outdoor activities, such as climbing, mountain biking, and kayaking.
- When planning a trip into the backcountry always devise a plan in advance on how to treat and evacuate all types of musculoskeletal injuries. This plan includes treatment plans, supplies, and how to evacuate a person should a significant injury occur.

Evacuation Guidelines

- Reasons for evacuating victims with musculoskeletal injuries from the wilderness include:
  - Sprains that are significant enough to prevent further activities in the wilderness.
  - Any victim who has loss of sensation or impaired circulation beyond the site of the injury.
  - All suspected fractures, whether open or closed should be evacuated. Certain fractures are considered life threatening:
    - Femur fracture
    - Pelvic fracture
    - Neck fracture
    - Spine fracture
  - Any individual who is unable to complete all predicted activities in the wilderness due to a sustained injury.

Questions

1. Which one of the following features defines an open fracture?
    a. Break in the skin (laceration) over the fracture site
    b. Loss of circulation beyond the wound
    c. Major deformity at the fracture site
    d. Severe uncontrolled pain

2. Life threatening fractures include all but which one of the following?
    a. Femur fracture
    b. Lower leg fracture
    c. Neck fracture
    d. Pelvis fracture

3. You are mountain biking when you come upon another rider who has fallen off his bike. He is holding his left shoulder with his right hand and is in a significant amount of pain around the left shoulder. After examining the victim, you are unsure as to whether he has a dislocation or a fracture. You should perform all of the following except:
    a. Apply ice to his shoulder
    b. Check for circulation to his left arm
    c. Pull on his arm in an attempt to reduce the potential dislocation
    d. Splint his arm with his elbow bent at 90 degrees

4. Which one of the following is a correct in terms of making a splint for a suspected forearm fracture that is closed?
    a. Have the splint immobilize the elbow and the wrist
    b. Have the splint immobilize the elbow only
    c. Have the splint immobilize the wrist only
    d. Have the splint immobilize the wrist, elbow and shoulder

ANSWERS
1. a 2. b 3. c 4. a

CHAPTER 7
Drowning and Water Safety

Objectives:
- Define the basic terms of drowning, the drowning process, and survival
- Be able to describe the mechanism of shallow water blackout
- Be able to describe what happens to the body when someone drowns
- To demonstrate the initial management of a victim of a drowning in the wilderness setting
- Be able to describe which patients require evacuation to a medical setting
- Be able to describe methods to prevent drowning

> ## Case 7.1
>
> An eighteen-year-old male falls out of a raft in a class IV rapid and is repeatedly pulled under the water as he fights his way through the rapids. He is pulled out of the water on the shore and is awake and alert. He is coughing vigorously and complains of shortness of breath and a full sensation in his chest. His past medical history is unremarkable.
> Vital signs: HR = 108, RR = 28.
>
> Physical examination is remarkable for respiratory distress with pulling in along his ribs. The remainder of his examination is normal.
>
> - What is the next step in the management of this patient?
> - Are there any other vital signs you would be interested in obtaining for this patient, if possible?
> - Does he require evacuation or can he stay in the backcountry with observation?

Background

Terminology
- **Drowning**: A process resulting in primary respiratory impairment from submersion / immersion in a liquid medium. The victim may live or die during or after this process.
- **The Drowning Process**: A continuum that begins when the victim's airway lies below the surface of liquid, usually water, preventing the victim from breathing air. A victim may be rescued during the drowning process and may not require intervention or may receive appropriate resuscitative measure.
- **Drowned**: refers to a person who dies from drowning
- **Survival**: Indicates that the victim remained alive after the submersion event and any subsequent problems that were caused by this event.

Shallow Water Blackout
- A special cause of drowning that occurs in people who hyperventilate before entering the water for an underwater swim.
- Hyperventilation significantly reduces the carbon dioxide level without increasing oxygen storage.
- The body uses a high carbon dioxide level in the blood as the marker of the need to breath.
- The vigorous underwater activity uses the available oxygen, causing low blood oxygen but before sufficient CO_2 accumulates to provide a stimulus to return to the surface. The patient loses consciousness due to the low oxygen and sustains a drowning event.

Drowning Statistics
- In many areas of the world, drowning is a leading cause of death, especially among young children.
- According to the World Health Organization, more than 500,000 deaths each year are due to drowning.
- Drowning is second only to motor vehicle accidents as the most common cause of accidental death in the United States
- Drowning mainly kills the young.
    - 64 percent of all victims are under age 30
    - 26 percent of all victims are under age 5
    - Most drownings occur in very young children with large numbers of deaths in 4 year old children, and in young adults and adolescents aged 15 to 24.
- Freshwater drowning, especially in pools, is more common than saltwater drowning. This includes coastal areas.

What happens in drowning?

General

- The basic problem in drowning is respiratory failure with low blood oxygen. This lack of oxygen can result in damage to the heart and brain.
- Older victims who are not immediately unconscious may initially panic and struggle in the water.
    - They will hold their breath and try to stay above the water surface.
    - Breath holding will occur under the water.
    - Eventually, a breaking point is reached and the body involuntarily breathes, even if the victim is under water.
- At the point of involuntary breathing, the victim inhales water into the lungs,

Organ System Effects

Lungs
- The lung is the primary organ injured by drowning.
- They become stiff and less able to expand as well as losing the ability to transmit oxygen into the blood.
- The symptoms can be mild to severe depending on the extent of the lung injury.
- Signs and symptoms:
    - Shortness of breath
    - Difficulty breathing
    - Cough
    - Wheezing

Heart
- Cardiac arrhythmias (irregular heart beat) are common in drowning incidents. However, these are usually due to the low blood oxygen levels.

Brain
- 12 to 27 percent of drowning victims sustain brain damage.
- Insults to the brain usually result from a lack of oxygen.
- Be concerned for cervical spine injuries when victims have been diving into pools or waters of an unknown depth.

Cold Water Drowning
- Hypothermia may be "protective" if it occurs before irreversible hypoxia and allow a drowning victim to recover with a better outcome. This occurs most commonly in children.
- However, most hypothermic drowning victims are cold from prolonged exposure and are simply dead.

Treatment

- Rapid but cautious rescue so that the rescuers do not become victims.
- The gold standard is immediate and aggressive initiation of rescue breathing.
- Remember that drowning victims often also have traumatic injuries. Remember to treat these problems and to protect the spine from further injury if there is any concern.
- CPR should be started on any patient with even a remote possibility of success.
    - Prompt initiation of rescue breathing increases survival.
    - Drowning victims with only respiratory arrest usually respond after a few rescue breaths.

- Interestingly, the Europeans Resuscitation Council recommends five initial rescue breaths instead of two (as recommended by the American Heart Association) because the initial ventilations can be more difficult to achieve in drowning victims.
  - If there is no response to the initial rescue breaths, the victims should be assumed to be in cardiac arrest and be taken as quickly as possible to dry land where effective CPR can be initiated.
  - Victims of cold-water submersion should ideally be warmed to before CPR is discontinued.
  - Victims of warm water submersion or those who have a normal body temperature and have CPR ongoing for 20 to 30 minutes without success may have CPR terminated.
- The Heimlich maneuver at one time was recommended by the American Red Cross and AHA. However, this technique is no longer recommended.
- If the person is unconscious but breathing, place them on their side in the recovery position in case they vomit.

Evacuation Guidelines

- All drowning victims should be evacuated as they may develop worsening symptoms over time.

Prevention

- Prevention is more important than any action one can take after a submersion incident has occurred.
- Alcohol should be avoided when participating in or supervising water activities.
- Everyone on a boat should always wear approved personal flotation devices that will support the person's head above water, even if the person becomes unconscious.
- Camp far enough away from water so that people, especially children, do not accidentally wander into the water.
- Anyone who works on or near the water should have swimming, rescue, and life-saving skills.
- Young children should always be supervised when around water.
  - A one-minute phone call or other distraction is all it takes for a child to become submerged.
  - Toddlers have drowned in toilets and small buckets of water.
  - Toddlers have drowned in bathtubs when left alone with older siblings to watch them without adult supervision.
- Patients with seizure disorders should always be supervised if swimming and should probably bathe in showers.
- Swimming pools:
  - These should be completely enclosed by a 5-foot fence with self-closing and self-latching locks.
  - This fence should also separate the pool from the house. This means that the pool should not be directly open to the back door of the house.
  - Appropriate life-saving equipment such as a pole to pull people to the side and personal flotation devices should be near the pool.
  - Owners of swimming pools should be trained in CPR.
  - Children whose families have a pool should take swimming lessons early.

Questions

1. **Which one of the following is the mechanism behind shallow water blackout?**
    a. Hyperventilation results in an increased blood oxygen level, causing one to lose the drive to surface to breathe
    b. Hyperventilation results in an increased blood carbon dioxide level, causing one to lose the drive to surface to breathe
    c. The oxygen level in the blood drops too low before one has the drive to surface to breathe due to the carbon dioxide level being too low
    d. Vigorous activity causes the carbon dioxide level to drop while under the water

2. **Which one of the following describes the basic pathophysiology of drowning?**
    a. Brain swelling due to excessive fluid intake
    b. Cardiac abnormalities from too much oxygen in the blood
    c. Lung injury due to stiff lungs and inability to absorb oxygen into the blood
    d. Respiratory difficulty due to pneumonia caused by bacteria in the aspirated water

3. **A 30-year-old male dives headfirst off a cliff into a lake. He surfaces within 5 seconds but is floating and appears to be unconscious. Which one of the following is the most likely etiology for his symptoms?**
    a. He hyperventilated before jumping in the water and suffered an arrest due to an increased blood carbon dioxide level
    b. He suffered a cardiac arrest due to the suddenness coldness of the water
    c. He suffered a cardiac arrest due to inhaling water
    d. He suffered a cervical injury with resultant paralysis by striking the bottom of the lake

4. **Which one of the following is <u>not</u> part of the management of the drowning victim in the field setting?**
    a. Heimlich maneuver to increase stomach emptying
    b. Immediate CPR if the patient is not breathing
    c. Stabilization of the cervical spine if there is concern of injury
    d. Thorough assessment of the respiratory system if the patient is awake

5. **Which one of the following is <u>not</u> a method to help prevent drowning?**
    a. All rafters should wear personal flotation devices
    b. Alcohol should be consumed in moderation when around the water
    c. Camp sites should be established far away from water, especially when children are present
    d. Those working around or on water should have CPR and water rescue skills

ANSWERS
1. c 2. c 3. c 4. a 5. b

CHAPTER 8

Lightning Injuries and Prevention

Objectives:
- Recognize when and where lightning is more likely to strike in relation to a storm
- Be able to describe the six mechanisms by which one may be struck by lightning
- Understand the concept of "reverse triage" in managing multiple casualties from a lightning strike
- Understand that all victims of a lightning strike should be evacuated as soon as possible from the wilderness
- Be able to list several methods to minimize the potential that one may be struck by lightning while in the wilderness

Case 8.1

A 23-year-old male is leaning against a vehicle when the large whip antenna is struck by lightning. He is thrown back from the vehicle and is slightly confused about what actually happened. On your evaluation, he is awake and alert. He remembers a large flash of light. The next thing he remembers is being on the ground 10 feet away from the vehicle. His physical examination is normal, with the exception of an unusual rash on his left chest (Figure 19.1).

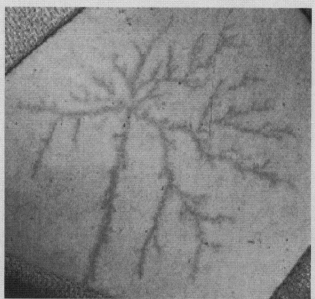

Figure 19.1 Rash on the Left Side of the Chest in Case 8.1

- What is the next step in the management of this victim?
- Are you at risk of electrical injury from a residual electrical charge if you touch him?
- Does he require evacuation to a hospital, or can he stay in the wilderness and continue his journey.

Types of Lightning Injuries

Direct strike

- The victim is struck directly by the bolt of lightning.
- This most commonly occurs to people who are caught in the open and are unable to find cover.

Side splash

- The lightning directly strikes another object such as a tree or building, but the current flow jumps from its original pathway onto the victim.
- This is the most common cause of lightning injury.
- Side splashes may also splash indoors from metal objects, such as plumbing and telephones.
- Splashes may occur from person to person when several people are standing close together.

Contact

- Contact exposure occurs when a person is holding onto or touching an object that is either directly hit or splashed by lightning.
- The current passes through the object to the victim.

Ground current or step voltage

- Ground current is produced when lightning strikes the ground or a nearby object and the current spreads through the ground.
- If a person has one foot closer to the strike, then a potential difference may exist between the two feet and the current will pass up one leg and down the other leg.
- This occurs because the body is of lower resistance than the ground.
- This is a common mechanism for several people being injured at the same time.

Injury by a weak upward streamer

- The electrical streamer heads upward into the sky but does not reach sky lightning, thus not completing a connection.
- The electrical charge passes over and through the involved individual but at a lesser energy than the amount from a direct strike from the sky.

Blunt trauma

- The injury occurs due to the impact of the concussive force of the strike itself, or due to being thrown because of the extreme nature of muscular contractions from the electrical charge.

Injuries Caused by Lightning

Heart
- The most common cause of death in a lightning victim is a lack of breathing or heart beat.
- A victim may suffer an initial cardiac arrest but recover his heartbeat in a period of seconds to minutes. However, if the victim stops breathing because of damage to the part of the brain that controls breathing (a very common occurrence), they may sustain a second cardiac arrest due to lack of oxygen from not breathing.
- The recovery of the drive to breathe usually occurs later than when the heart starts beating on its own. That is why it is important to anticipate the need to continue rescue breathing for victims even if they recover a pulse.

Brain
- Bleeding in the brain can occur from a current that traverses the brain.
- Victims who sustain burns to the head are four times more likely to die than those without cranial burns.
- Seizures may occur after a lightning strike.
- Confusion and loss of memory are very common.
- Long-term effects may include memory impairment, difficulty concentrating, sleep disturbances, and personality changes.
- Temporary paralysis of the upper or lower extremities can occur.

Respiratory system
- The victim may stop breathing from the lightning strike due to damage to the part of the brain which controls breathing (i.e. brain stem).
- The victim may sustain bruises to the lung and cough up bloody sputum.

Skin
- Contrary to popular myth and what is seen in cartoons, deep burns are unusual after lightning injury. At the most, some minor partial thickness burns may occur from superheated metal objects in contact with the skin.
- Often there are no burns.
- There are four types of common skin effects:
  - *Ferning* (Figure 19.1): Also called "feathering" or "Lichtenberg figures". These are not actual burns, but an unusual pattern that occurs due to the electron shower that courses over the skin surface.
  - *Linear burns*: These burns occur from steam production from sweat or water that instantaneously heats and evaporates on the victim due to the increased temperatures associated with the lightning strike.
  - *Punctate burns*: These are multiple, closely spaced, but discrete circular burns that individually range from a few millimeters to a centimeter in thickness.
  - *Thermal burns*: These are regular thermal burns that occur when a victim is wearing a metal object, such as a belt buckle or necklace, which heats up due to the electrical current traversing it. There may also be thermal burns if clothing ignites.

Musculoskeletal system
- Fractures and dislocations may occur due to intense muscular contractions or from the trauma of being thrown.

Ear
- Temporary deafness can occur due to the intense noise and shock wave.
- 30% to 50% of victims rupture one or both ear drums.
- Victims who were using a conventional (wired) telephone at the time of the strike are at high risk for hearing injuries, especially if there is a side splash into a dwelling through the telephone.

Eye
- Temporary blindness of both eyes may occur, but this is usually only temporary.
- Multiple types of internal eye damage can occur.
- Fixed dilated pupils occur as well, so do not rely on this as an absolute sign of death in a victim of lightning strike.

Signs of Lightning Injury

Single Victim
- Identification of a victim of a lightning strike is readily made if the strike was witnessed.
- In the case of the unwitnessed strike victim, clues that can assist you include environmental conditions, such as a recent thunderstorm or lightning.
- If the victim displays confusion and amnesia, as well as prominent physical findings such as ruptured ear drums and the classic skin finding of ferning, these findings assist in the diagnosis.

Multiple Victims
- The typical description of a multiple casualty lightning strike is one of a sudden flash of bright light followed closely by a loud boom and then chaos.
- There will likely be several people who are walking around but are confused. There will be people who are lying on the ground but are moving or breathing on their own. These first two groups of people do not require immediate attention.
- The final group of casualties may include one to several people who are unconscious, not breathing, and do not have a pulse. This final group is the one that requires immediate attention. The fact that you are first treating persons who appear dead is called "reverse triage." The reason for this reverse triage is due to the fact that victims who are awake or breathing have survived the most immediate and potentially critical injury, which is cardiac and respiratory arrest.

- Victims who are not breathing and have no pulse require CPR. Some of these victims will regain a heartbeat and respiratory drive, but it may take up to 10-15 minutes before this occurs. Performing CPR on these victims can save their lives if their heart and brain are not too severely damaged.
- In attempting to decide on which victims you should start the CPR, remember that those with head burns are four times more likely to die than persons without head burns.

Treatment of Lightning Injury

- Perform reverse triage and initiate CPR on victims who are not breathing and have no pulse before caring for those who have signs of life.
- Victims without spontaneous breathing or heartbeat may recover their heartbeat and will require assisted breathing until their respiratory drive returns. Breathing for these victims may prevent secondary cardiac arrest due to lack of oxygen.
- Call for evacuation to the closest medical facility.
- Stabilization and splinting of fractures and dislocations and spinal precautions should be performed as determined by the secondary assessment.
- Lightning does not leave a residual electrical charge on a victim of a strike. There is no need to be concerned about getting shocked by rescuing a person who has been struck by lightning.

Prevention

When thunder roars, go indoors

- The previous rule used to be the 30-30 rule where one should seek shelter if the time between seeing the lightning and hearing the thunder is 30 seconds or less.
- That rule has been replaced by an easier rule to remember: "When thunder roars go indoors". If you hear thunder, then you should seek shelter. This is based on the fact that the distances that sound travels are well within the distance of a lightning strike. Furthermore, you may miss lightning because it is hidden by the clouds or other terrain.

Seek shelter in a substantial building or in an all-metal vehicle

- Small shelters, such as golf carts, buses, and rain shelters, may increase a person's risk of being struck due to side splash as the lightning flows over the shelter.
- All metal vehicles are safe because the metal will diffuse the current around the occupants to the ground. A convertible automobile is not a safe alternative. It is a myth that the rubber tires on a vehicle provide insulation.

If you are caught in a storm outside without a safe building or vehicle:

- Stay away from metal objects and items that are taller than you.
- Avoid areas near power lines, pipelines, ski lifts, and other large steel objects.
- Do not stand near or under tall isolated trees, hilltops, or at a lookout or other exposed area.
- In a forest, seek a low area under a growth of saplings or small trees. Seeking a clearing free of trees makes a person the tallest object in the clearing.
- If you are in a group of people, spread far apart so that a single lightning strike will not take out the entire group.
- If on the water, seek the shore and avoid being the tallest object near a large body of water.

- The more dangerous times for a severe lightning strike are before the storm appears and after it has passed.
- Lightning does strike twice in the same place - all the time.
- If you are totally in the open, stay far away from single trees to avoid lightning splashes and ground current. A good position is to squat down with your knees fully bent and your feet together. This way a current will go through your feet and not through your heart. You can also sit cross-legged if you want. Try to cover your ears so that thunder will not damage your hearing.

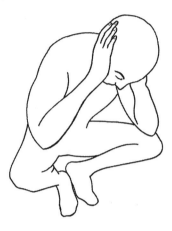

Figure 19.2 Lightning Position

If indoors:

Avoid open doors, windows, fireplaces, and metal objects such as sinks. Plug in electrical appliances.

Evacuation Guidelines

- Any victim of a lightning strike should be evacuated as soon as possible.
- Even if the individual does not have any overt evidence of physical injury, there is a high likelihood of some sort of injury that is not served best by staying in the wilderness.

Questions

1. **What is the most dangerous time to be struck by lightning in relation to the storm?**
    a. The very first time you hear thunder
    b. In the middle of the storm, when the rain is hardest
    c. The period of time right before the storm actually hits
    d. You are at the same risk regardless of the stage of the storm

2. **In which one of the following situations is somebody least likely to get injured by lightning?**
    a. Sitting inside a rain shelter that is open from the front on a golf course
    b. Sitting under a large tree that provides protection from the rain
    c. Sitting in an all-metal automobile with the windows rolled up
    d. Standing upright in the middle of an open field

3. **A 30-year-old male is struck by lightning and is not breathing. Which one of the following is correct in regards to the management of this victim?**
    a. CPR is not necessary as his heart will resume beating on its own
    b. CPR is not helpful as his heart likely sustained irreversible damage
    c. CPR should be initiated until he begins breathing on his own, then you may stop
    d. CPR should not be initiated, because the victim may carry a residual charge from the lightning and thereby injure the rescuer

4. **You observe lightning strike a large group of people with the following casualties:**
    1. Awake, alert, and sitting up with obvious dislocated shoulder
    2. Awake, moaning, and confused
    3. Unconscious, not breathing, no evidence of injury
    4. Unconscious, not breathing, obvious burn to the head and face
    5. Unconscious, breathing on own

    Which is the correct order that you should care for these victims?

    a. 1, 2, 5, 4, 3
    b. 2, 5, 4, 3, 1
    c. 3, 4, 5, 2, 1
    d. 4, 3, 5, 2, 1
    e. 5, 3, 4, 2, 1

5. **Which one of the following is a method to minimize being struck by lightning?**
    a. If caught in the open, squat down with your feet together
    b. Seek shelter under the largest tree out in the open, ensuring you are leaning against it
    c. Lay down on your back if you are caught in the open
    d. Seek shelter when you see lightning and hear thunder within 10 seconds
    e. Sit under large electrical towers because they are grounded and protected from lightning

ANSWERS
1. c 2. c 3. c 4. c 5. a

CHAPTER 9

Head Trauma and Spine Injuries

Objectives:
- Know basic brain anatomy
- Be able to recognize common head injuries
- Be able to treat common head injuries
- Know basic spine anatomy
- Know common mechanisms of how the spinal cord is injured
- Know initial treatment for spinal cord injures

> ## Case 9.1
>
> During a hike, a 20-year-old female falls off of a small boulder and hits her head. She loses consciousness for a brief moment. She awakes and is bleeding from the side of her head. She also scraped her back.
>
> - What is the initial management of this patient?
> - What are the major concerns to watch for?
> - How do you treat the head wound?

Head Trauma

Scalp Laceration

- Scalp lacerations are common and when they occur, they will typically bleed profusely.
  - The bleeding is because of the blood-rich nature of the scalp.
  - Scalp blood vessels typically do not constrict rapidly to slow bleeding.
- The best was to stop the bleeding is with direct pressure from a bulky dressing.
- Clean the wound thoroughly with water when possible.
- Clip hair to visualize wound if needed.
  - However, do not shave the hair, as this may increase the risk of infection
- Closure
  - Butterfly bandages or skin closure strips work well.
  - Apply the strips perpendicular to wound.
  - Pull wound together, but not too tight.
  - Dress with antibiotic ointment and sterile gauze.
  - Monitor for signs and symptoms of infection.

Concussions

- Patients with mild head injuries typically have concussions.
- A concussion is defined as injury to the brain without any evidence of structural alteration.
- Typical symptoms include:
  - Confusion
  - Loss of memory (amnesia)
  - Dizziness
  - Nausea/vomiting
  - Disorientation
  - Slurred speech
  - Loss of consciousness
  - Very emotional
  - Headache
- If a concussion is suspected then those displaying persistent vomiting, severe headache, amnesia or loss of consciousness should be evacuated.

Skull Fracture

- Skull fractures may occur with head injuries.
- While the skull is tough and provides excellent protection for the brain, a severe impact or blow can result in fracture of the skull.
- It may be accompanied by injury to the brain.
- The brain can be affected directly by damage to the nervous system tissue and bleeding. The brain can also be affected indirectly by blood clots that form under the skull and then compress the underlying brain tissue.

Signs and symptoms

- Decreased level of consciousness
- Deformity (often a depression) at the injury site
- Possible "Raccoon eyes" (black and blue discoloration around eyes)
- Possible Battle sign (black and blue discoloration behind and below the ears)
- Seizures
- Clear fluid (spinal fluid) leaking from nose or ears

Treatment

- Do not attempt to stop the flow of fluid from nose/ears.
- Impaled objects should NOT be removed.
- Stabilize object in place with large bulky dressings.
- Patient should be evacuated immediately.

Closed Head Injury

- This is from a violent impact to the head that does not fracture the skull.
- Such trauma may involve a period of unconsciousness.
- Bleeding inside the head results in increased intracranial pressure (ICP) that can result in permanent brain damage or death.
- Physical findings:
  - Headache
  - Increased blood pressure
  - Visual disturbances
  - Excessive sleepiness
  - Protracted nausea and vomiting
  - Loss of balance (ataxia)
  - Seizures
  - Unequal pupils
  - Rigid body postures

Treatment of Head Injuries

- No loss of consciousness
  - Mostly stable with a lower chance of serious problems
  - Monitor patient for 24 hours at a minimum
  - Evacuate if signs of serious brain damage develop
- Momentary loss of consciousness / "dazed"
  - Monitor closely for 24 hours
  - Wake patient every couple of hours to monitor and to ensure that they are acting normal and answering questions appropriately
  - Evacuate if any signs of brain injury occur, such as confusion, memory problems, severe headache or just not appearing to be themselves

- Loss of consciousness
  - Evacuate immediately
- Determining when to evacuate may be a difficult decision
  - If you evacuate anybody knocked unconscious, you will be acting responsibly
  - If the patient experiences only a momentary loss of consciousness and responds immediately to verbal stimuli and has no signs of brain injury they are probably okay to stay in the wilderness
- Do not give painkilling medications
  - They may mask the signs and symptoms of a serious brain injury and make it difficult to diagnosis
  - Aspirin and NSAIDs (including ibuprofen and naproxen) may increase bleeding in the brain so avoid these medicines
- If you have to leave the patient alone for any reason
  - Ensure that the patient doesn't lose their airway
  - Roll patient on his/her side

Spine Injuries

- Spinal cord trauma is damage to the spinal cord.
- It may result from direct injury to the cord itself or indirectly from disease of the surrounding bones, tissues, or blood vessels.

Anatomy of the Spinal Cord and the Spine

- Cervical (neck) vertebrae – there are 7 of them – these are numbered from the top C1 – C7
  - These are the least protected of all the vertebrae.
  - They are the most prone to serious injury.
- Thoracic (chest) vertebrae – there are 12 of them – these are numbered from the top T1 – T12
  - These are attached to ribs protecting the organs of the chest.
  - These are protected by the back muscles.
- Lumbar (lower back) vertebrae – there are 5 of them – these are numbered from the top L1 – L5
  - These are the strongest of the vertebrae
  - The surrounding muscles are prone to injury from lifting and twisting.
- Sacral vertebrae
  - Fused and attached to pelvic girdle
- Coccyx – the tailbone
- The spinal cord passes through the middle of each vertebra (spinal bone)
- There are discs of cartilage between each vertebra which allow movement and help absorb shock. In time, these tend to degenerate.
- Nerve roots branch out from between the vertebrae and send peripheral nerves to the rest of the body.

Mechanism of Spine Injuries

- Excessive flexion (bending the head forward as if looking down to the ground) – diver hits the bottom of a shallow pond
- Excessive extension (bending the head backwards as if looking up at the sky) – whiplash in car accident
- Compression (pushing the spine bones together forcefully) – climber falls and lands sitting
- Distraction (pulling the spine apart forcefully by pulling on each end) – hanging
- Excessive rotation (turning too hard to one side) – ski injury

Assessment of Spinal Injuries

- Treat all unconscious trauma patients as if they have a spinal injury.
- Initial assessment – is the patient breathing?
  - If a patient has a spinal cord injury above C4 – they will likely not be breathing.
  - Patients with spinal cord injuries between C4 and T1 may result in "belly breathing"
- Vital Signs – is the patient in neurogenic shock?
  - Loss of control over the dilation and constriction of blood vessels due to nerve damage.
  - Warm and flushed (from dilated blood vessels) below the site of injury

Spinal Cord Injury – Signs and Symptoms

- The symptoms vary from patient to patient and also depend upon the mechanism of injury (MOI)
- A person who falls from a 30-foot cliff is more likely to have significant trauma then someone who slips off a chair.
- If any trauma to the spinal cord is suspected either from the mechanism of injury or from the examination, be aggressive in the management of the patient.
- There are some typical signs:
  - Labored breathing
  - Altered sensation such as numbness, tingling or burning pain
  - Weakness or paralysis
  - Pain and/or tenderness along the spine
  - Obvious evidence of injury to the spine (cuts, punctures, bruises)

Examination of the Spine
- Do not allow the patient to move.
- Examination
  - Carefully roll patient onto his/her side
  - Use 3-4 rescuers to keep the patient's spine immobilized
- Palpate every vertebra but stop if the patient reports intense pain.
- Look for signs of a back injury.

Clearing a C-Spine
- There are situations in the wilderness when it is important to determine if the cervical spine is free from injury.
- This might be seen when evacuation makes it essential.
- So, when a significant mechanism of injury is present, a cervical spine is determined to be stable if:
  - There is no bony tenderness in the midline of the cervical vertebrae.
  - There patient is not intoxicated
  - The patient is alert and oriented to person, place, time, and event
  - There are no new neurological complaints or problems (e.g. tingling, numbness or weakness in the limbs or body).
  - There are no painful distracting injuries (e.g., long bone fracture)
- A mnemonic to help remember this is the absence of all of these:
  - **C** – Cervical midline tenderness
  - **S** – Sensory-motor deficit (numbness/weakness)
  - **P** – Pain that is bad enough to distract from neck pain
  - **I** – Intoxication from alcohol or other drugs
  - **N** – Neurologic loss (loss of alertness)
  - **E** – Events (sufficient mechanism to cause neck injury)

Treatment
- Remember is it always better to over-treat suspected spinal cord injuries rather than to undertreat.
- Start with manually stabilizing the head and cervical spine
  - Keep the patient as still as possible
  - Assure an airway (use jaw thrust if needed)
- Check for circulation, sensation, and motion in the extremities
- Apply a cervical collar
- Move patient to a backboard or rigid litter

Evacuation Guidelines

- Suspected skull fracture
- Penetrating head wound
- If a concussion is suspected then those displaying persistent vomiting, severe headache, memory loss, loss of consciousness
- Any concern for a brain injury, regardless of what may be causing it
- Anyone suspected of a spinal fracture
- Anyone suspected of having a spinal cord injury

Questions

- **Bleeding from head wounds should be treated with a bulky dressing because?**
    a. Bulky material is found more readily in the back country
    b. It will help prevent bone fragments from pressing into the brain in the event that there is a skull fracture
    c. This type of dressing will absorb blood more readily

- **What is the Battle sign?**
    a. Swelling and black and blue around the eyes
    b. Redness and discoloration behind the ears
    c. Clear fluid and blood coming from the nose

- **Which is not included in the mnemonic C-SPINE when ruling out a cervical spine injury?**
    o C   – Cerebral spinal fluid in the ears or nose
    o S   – Sensory-motor deficit (numbness/weakness)
    o P   – Pain that is bad enough to distract from neck pain
    o I   – Intoxication from alcohol or other drugs
    o N   – Neurologic loss (loss of alertness)
    o E   – Events (sufficient mechanism to cause neck injury)

- **Above which vertebrae is it likely that a spinal injury will result in an inability to breathe?**
    o L4
    o T3
    o C7
    o C4

- **True/False: An unconscious trauma patient can be ruled out of a spinal cord injury.**

ANSWERS
1. b 2. b 3. a 4. d 5. f

CHAPTER 10

Medical Problems in the Wilderness

Objectives:
- Evaluate and determine the need for evacuation of patients with chest pain in the wilderness
- Evaluate and determine the need for evacuation of patients with shortness of breath in the wilderness
- Understand and treat neurological problems in the wilderness
- Understand and treat issues with diabetes in the wilderness
- Recognize and treat allergic reactions
- Evaluate abdominal pain and know when patients need to be evacuated from the wilderness
- Describe various methods that may be used to prevent the most common infectious diseases in wilderness travel
- Identify when a patient with an infectious disease must be evacuated from the wilderness

Chest Pain Related Emergencies

> ### Case 10.1
>
> A 56-year-old man is on day four of a seven-day rafting trip. He is paddling a raft through a calm stretch of water. He begins to experience chest pain that spreads to his left shoulder. The pain is significant enough that he has to pull over to the shore. He describes pressure in his chest as well.
>
> - What questions should you ask this patient?
> - What are some life-threatening causes of chest pain?
> - Does he require evacuation or can he stay on the trip?

Chest pain can occur for many different reasons. Pain related to the heart, lungs, stomach, bones and muscles of the chest wall can all cause chest pain. The primary goal of the wilderness medicine provider is to try and determine if the cause of the chest pain is life threatening, and thus requires evacuation. This can be very difficult, even for a physician in a hospital setting. In general, the wilderness first responder should always practice the "better safe than sorry" philosophy when it comes to evaluating chest pain.

Heart-Related Chest Pain

There are several conditions that can cause chest pain related to the heart. Infection, trauma, heart muscle inflammation, and heart attacks are all serious causes of chest pain. A patient is more likely to have chest pain related to a heart attack or other life-threatening condition if they have any of the following conditions:

- Age > 50
- Medical history of high blood pressure, diabetes, or high cholesterol
- Previous history of heart problems
- Uses tobacco of any kind
- Significantly overweight

Always use the SAMPLE and COLDERR acronyms discussed in the patient assessment chapter when obtaining a medical history and characterizing the patient's pain. If a patient's cause of chest pain is related to the heart, they may complain of one or more of the following symptoms:

- Onset with activity: often the pain will start with activity, where the heart is beating faster and using more oxygen.
- Chest pain or pressure: this is often described as a squeezing or tightness, often with a clenched fist over the chest. The pain is usually in the center of the chest, but may radiate to the left arm, jaw, neck or back.
- Shortness of breath: especially with activity (even light activity).
- Nausea or vomiting: this is a frequent symptom if the patient and the heart are strained.
- Dizziness and sweating

Other Causes of Chest Pain

There are many other life-threatening causes of chest pain for which further description is beyond the scope of this text. In general, any of the following associated historical features and symptoms should make the wilderness responder suspicious of a life-threatening cause of pain:
- History of blood clots in the legs or lungs
- Difficulty breathing with activity or at rest that is worse than what the patient typically experiences
- Severe uncontrolled chest pain after several episodes of vomiting
- Associated fever, sweating, or lightheadedness
- Severe tearing pain that spreads to the back

Treatment

- Rest is the key to reducing stress on the heart muscle.
- If a patient has a history of heart-related chest pain and carries medications for a heart condition (such as nitroglycerin), they can take them as previously instructed by their physician.
- Given time and rest, patients may be able to hike slowly downhill, but do not allow them to exert themselves if the pain is recurrent.
- If a patient has any concerning historical features or symptoms, they should be evacuated.

The diagnosis of heart-related chest pain is very complex, especially without the tools found in a hospital setting. A patient can still be having a heart attack or other life-threatening condition, even if they do not have any of the risk factors or symptoms listed above. IF IN DOUBT, always err on the side of rapid evacuation to emergency medical treatment.

Respiratory Emergencies

Case 10.2

A 22-year-old female begins to have difficulty breathing while hiking on a trip in Nepal. She is an asthmatic and carries asthma medication with her. You are four walking days from any city.

- What can this person do to help her own condition?
- What are some ways to help improve her shortness of breath?
- At what point should she be evacuated?

Shortness of Breath

Individuals can experience shortness of breath for many reasons in the wilderness, including asthma, pulmonary embolism, allergic reactions, pneumonia, emphysema, and high altitude pulmonary edema. These causes can be difficult to distinguish from one another, especially in the wilderness. The primary goal of the wilderness provider is not to determine the exact cause of a patient's shortness of breath, but more to give the patient some relief and determine whether or not the individual needs rapid evacuation. The following historical features and symptoms are concerning and are more likely to result in evacuation from the backcountry:

- History of emphysema or COPD (chronic obstructive pulmonary disease)
- Worsening shortness of breath with activity (worse than the individual typically has with activity)
- Signs of a respiratory infection such as fever, chills, and productive cough
- Chest pain associated with shortness of breath
- Coughing up blood and shortness of breath
- Severe asthma attack not responding to the patient's previously prescribed medications

Treatment

- Place the victim in a position that makes breathing as easy as possible.
- Minimize the patient's activities/exertion.
- Have the individual use any medications they have been previously prescribed for the condition (i.e. inhalers for asthma, etc.).
- If the symptoms do not resolve after a brief rest period, the patient should be evacuated.
- If the symptoms resolve, but then continue to recur despite multiple rest periods and treatment, the individual should be evacuated.
- Consider an infectious process such as pneumonia as the etiology of the symptoms.

Neurologic Emergencies

Case 10.3

While in camp, a 44-year-old female begins to have a seizure on day three of a nine-day trip to the Grand Canyon on the Colorado River. She has never had seizures before.

- What are some features of a true seizure?
- What should be done for this patient during the seizure?
- Does she require evacuation?

Seizures

Seizures can occur because of a seizure disorder or develop due to a recent injury or illness. Patients with known seizure disorders typically take medications to prevent them from occurring. A true generalized seizure typically has the following features:

- A sensation prior to the seizure where the patient may describe a sick feeling, an odd taste or strange smell
- Generalized shaking of the entire body
- Loss of bowel or bladder control
- Inability to speak or consciously control seizure activity
- A period of confusion after the seizure, often lasting 30 minutes to an hour

A seizure in a person without a seizure disorder can occur for many reasons, including the following:

- Low blood sugar
- Head injury
- Infection of the brain
- Exposure to some type of toxic substance (poison)
- Stroke

Treatment

The primary role of the wilderness provider is to protect a patient while they are actively seizing. Methods to help prevent secondary injury in a patient having a seizure include the following:

- A seizure must run its course once it has begun. While the wilderness provider cannot stop the seizure, the patient must be prevented from hurting him/herself.
- If the patient begins to turn blue or appears to be choking, attempt to open the airway using the methods discussed in the patient assessment chapter.
- Do not try and hold a patient down or restrain them unless they are in immediate danger of hurting themselves, such as on a narrow trail bordered by a cliff.
- Move objects away from the patient and move the patient away from cliffs, water, or other hazards.
- A patient cannot swallow their tongue, so do NOT try to put anything into the mouth.
- Once a patient stops seizing, they should be rolled onto their side (assuming they have not fallen a significant distance and there is no concern for neck injury) with their head supported by a pack or some folded clothing.
- Check the patient from head to toe for injuries related to their seizure after they recover.
- All patients with a seizure must be evacuated.
- If the seizure fails to stop or continues to recur for 15 minutes, the patient is considered to be in "status epilepticus" and will likely not stop without some type of intervention. DO NOT wait this long to arrange immediate evacuation from the wilderness. This is a true emergency because prolonged or recurrent seizures prevent adequate breathing and can lead to permanent brain injury.

In a person with a known seizure disorder, it is recommended that they be seizure free for at least six months before entering the backcountry. Another group member should always carry an extra set of the individual's anti-seizure medicines in case of loss or ruin of the primary set.

Stroke

A stroke is an injury to an area of the brain, usually from lack of blood flow. Signs and symptoms vary depending on the part of the brain that is affected. A stroke may lead to one or more of the following symptoms:

- Alteration in mental status (confusion, stupor, semi-consciousness, unconsciousness)
- Decrease in muscle strength – usually on one side
- Unsteady gait
- Numbness – usually on one side
- One-sided facial paralysis or facial drooping
- Garbled, slurred, or confused speech
- Blurred vision

Treatment

Strokes can be debilitating and life threatening. There is not much that can or should be done in the backcountry.

- Make the patient as comfortable as possible. Patients who are unable to assume a comfortable position should be placed on the weak or paralyzed side to protect their airway.
- Evacuate as soon as possible.

Diabetic Emergencies

> ## Case 10.4
>
> While hiking in the backcountry with a number of scouts, you are called to examine a 14-year-old boy who is becoming unresponsive. He is a known diabetic and had a tag around his neck that indicates this. It is presumed that his blood sugars are falling.
>
> - What are some other symptoms of low blood sugar?
> - What is the next step in managing this patient?
> - What are the reasons that his blood sugars would be so low, and how could this be avoided?
> - Does he require evacuation?

Diabetes

The two primary emergencies that can arise in diabetics are very high and very low blood sugar. Diabetic emergencies are common in the outdoor setting where diabetics frequently exert themselves too much, don't stay well hydrated, and are not as careful about their food intake.

Symptoms of **low blood sugar** include the following:

- Rapid onset of confusion, irritability, or combativeness
- Hunger
- Pale, sweaty skin
- Loss of coordination, tremors, slurred speech
- Generalized weakness
- Headache, dizziness, and possible seizures

Symptoms of **high blood sugar** include the following:

- Very slow onset of confusion and irritability
- Hunger and thirst, frequent urination
- Headache
- Blurred vision
- Nausea and vomiting
- Fruity smelling breath and urine

Treatment
The treatment for **low blood sugar** includes:

- Sugar – any form of sugar will be sufficient, including candy, sports drinks, starchy foods, etc.
- If the patient is unconscious, sugar (in any form) can be rubbed carefully onto the gums.
- This is a true medical emergency that needs treatment in the backcountry setting.
- Evacuation should be considered for all patients unless they are cleared by a medical provider.

The treatment for **high blood sugar** includes:

- If the patient is comfortable managing mild elevations in their blood sugar using previous recommendations by their physician, that is fine. Ensure they are monitoring their sugar closely. If there is no significant change after several hours, the patient may need to be evacuated.

- Make sure the individual consumes lots of fluids. When blood sugar is high, the patient will urinate often, potentially leading to dehydration. Do not hydrate with only water. Alternate with very diluted sports drinks to help replace important electrolytes. The small amount of sugar found in diluted sports drinks will not make a significant impact on high blood sugar levels.

Allergic Reactions and Anaphylaxis

> **Case 10.5**
>
> You are biking on a trail east of a small city. You come across a 17-year-old female who is on the ground with a number of people gathered around her. She is having difficulty breathing and states she was stung by a bee while riding. She has a history of severe allergies to bee stings.
>
> - What is the most likely diagnosis of this patient?
> - What medicines should this patient receive?
> - Does she require evacuation?

Types of Reaction

There are two main types of allergic reactions: local and general.

Local
Local allergic reactions are characterized by these symptoms:
- Swollen and reddened area(s) of the skin
- Itchy (and sometimes painful) area(s) of the skin

General
Generalized allergic reactions many have the same symptoms as the local reaction in addition to any combination of the following:
- Hives
- Swelling to the face, arms or legs
- Nausea and vomiting
- Diarrhea

Any of these may begin minutes to hours after the exposure to the offending agent. Generalized reactions may progress to a condition called anaphylaxis, which is a life-threatening emergency. Symptoms of anaphylaxis include any of the above in addition to the following:

- Shortness of breath and wheezing
- Lightheadedness
- Swelling of the tongue and lips, airway constriction
- Confusion
- Tightness in the chest
- Loss of consciousness

Treatment

Local reactions:

- Cold packs may alleviate some of the irritation.
- Scratching should be minimized as it may open the area up to infection.
- Topical corticosteroids such as hydrocortisone cream can be helpful in relieving the symptoms.
- Over-the-counter antihistamines such as diphenhydramine (Benadryl) may be useful but can also cause drowsiness.

Generalized reactions:

- If it is known what the patient is allergic to, they should be removed from the source immediately.
- If over-the-counter diphenhydramine is available, it should be administered immediately. This may slow/prevent the anaphylactic reaction.
- If any respiratory symptoms are present, an EpiPen® or equivalent epinephrine auto injector should be administered. The wilderness medicine guide should be prepared to administer this medication if it is available.
- Any patient with symptoms of anaphylaxis should be evacuated, even if they improve with initial treatment.

Prevention

- If a member of the group entering the backcountry has a known severe allergy to something that they may be exposed to while in the wilderness, they must carry an epinephrine auto injector and diphenhydramine.
- Epinephrine auto injectors can be obtained by the individual with allergies from their physician prior to entering the backcountry.

Abdominal Emergencies

Case 10.6

You are on a multi-day hike in the wilderness with several people. One member of your party, a 22-year-old female, starts complaining of some lower abdominal pain. She denies fever and constipation, but does state some nausea. When asked about her last menstrual period, she states she "always has irregular periods." She wants to continue hiking but says the pain seems to be getting worse.

- What concerning features does this patient present with?
- What easy-to-carry test might be helpful in this case?
- Should this patient be evacuated or would observation be prudent?

Abdominal Pain

The exact cause of abdominal pain can be difficult to determine, especially in the backcountry setting. There are many life-threatening causes as well as many benign causes of abdominal pain. In general, certain features of a patient complaining of abdominal pain should alert the wilderness provider to a possibly serious cause:

- Pain with fever and chills
- Pain with vomiting
- Worse pain with movement (as opposed to no change in pain with position changes or walking)
- Pain in a pregnant female
- Pain in a female with unknown pregnancy status
- Blood in the stool, urine, or vomit
- Prolonged pain after trauma to the abdomen
- History of multiple previous abdominal surgeries
- History of previous ectopic pregnancy (pregnancy outside the uterus)

Common Causes in the Wilderness:
- Food poisoning (gastroenteritis)
- Dehydration leading to constipation
- Constipation
- Kidney stones
- Gallstones

Treatment

The primary goal of the wilderness provider is to make the patient comfortable and to determine if the patient should be evacuated.

Prevention

In general, it is difficult to "prevent" most causes of abdominal pain in the wilderness. Some things that can be done to help prevent an unnecessary evacuation include the following:

- Use appropriate water filtration devices. Contaminated water can lead to abdominal pain, vomiting and diarrhea.
- Maintain adequate hydration, and carry appropriate foods or medications to prevent constipation. Severe constipation can cause abdominal pain and may mimic more severe causes of pain.

General Evacuation Guidelines

Evacuate if abdominal pain is accompanied by one of the following conditions:
- Severe pain
- The pain persists for longer than 24 hours.
- Blood appears in the vomit, feces, or urine.
- The pain is associated with a fever.
- The pain is associated with pregnancy.
- The patient is unable to drink or eat.

Prevention of Infectious Diseases

Proper hygiene and sanitation practices are essential in preventing infectious diseases of the GI tract. The wilderness traveler must be vigilant to ensure that food and water do not become contaminated. The following guidelines are recommended:

Diet

- Wash hands thoroughly with soap or hand disinfectant before preparing and eating meals.
- Cooking and eating utensils should be cleaned with boiling water or bleach solution prior to each use.
- Avoid raw or undercooked meat, fish, and seafood.
- When traveling internationally, avoid street vendors, raw vegetables, and fresh salads.
- Avoid unpasteurized milk, cheese, and other dairy products.
- Peeled fruits and vegetables are generally safe.
- Do not rinse food in water that is not disinfected.

Water

- Use appropriate methods of water treatment.
- When traveling internationally, avoid tap water and ice cubes made from untreated water.
- Purchase name brand bottled water, and always check the seal prior to drinking.

When to Evacuate

- Any patient with moderate to severe abdominal pain that does not improve over 12-24 hours should be evacuated.
- Patients unable to take sufficient oral rehydration fluids for more than 24 hours should be evacuated.
- Anyone experiencing mental status changes, signs of significant dehydration, vomiting blood, or copious bloody stools should be evacuated immediately.
- Patients with diarrhea (especially containing blood or accompanied by fever or significant pain) who do not respond to appropriate antibiotic therapy in 24-48 hours should be evacuated.

General Evacuation Guidelines

Allergy Problems
Patients with symptoms of anaphylaxis or severe generalized allergic reaction should be evacuated for further medical evaluation.

Chest Pain
Patients with concerning historical features or symptoms as listed above should be evacuated for further medical evaluation. If there is any doubt, the patient should be evacuated.

Diabetic Emergencies
- Patients with high blood sugar should be evacuated if treatment is not working.
- Patients with low blood sugar should be evaluated for evacuation based on effectiveness of treatment and patient's wishes.

Neurologic Emergencies
- Evacuate any patient suffering a stroke, a TIA (minor stroke), or a new seizure.
- A significant change in mental status should lead to patient evacuation.

Shortness of Breath
- Patients complaining of shortness of breath with concerning historical features or symptoms, or those who do not improve with a brief period of rest should be evacuated immediately.
- Patients with known asthma need to be evacuated if their symptoms are not easily controlled with their own medications.

Abdominal Pain
- Severe pain
- Pain lasting longer than 24 hours
- Blood appears in the vomit, feces, or urine.
- The pain is associated with a fever.
- The pain is associated with pregnancy.
- The patient is unable to drink or eat.

Questions

1. **A member of your hiking party approaches you and states he is having some chest pain. Which of the following would not be a major concerning feature of his pain?**
    a. History of diabetes
    b. Associated shortness of breath
    c. The patient is 22-years-old
    d. The pain gets worse with exertion

2. **Which of the following patients with a history of asthma should be evacuated?**
    a. 33-year-old female whose symptoms resolve with a single use of her inhaler and do not recur
    b. 24-year-old female who forgot her inhaler on a day hike but is not having symptoms
    c. 37-year-old male on a multi-day rafting trip with wheezing, fever, and productive cough whose asthma symptoms do not fully respond to his inhaler
    d. 18-year-old male who uses his inhaler twice in one day during a multi-day hike

3. **While taking a break on a long single-track mountain bike course, your friend begins to have a seizure. He has never had seizures before as far as you know. Which of the following should NOT be performed during his seizure:**
    a. Avoid holding him down
    b. Clear the immediate area around him
    c. Placing objects in the patient's mouth
    d. Roll him on his side after the seizure has finished

4. **Common symptoms of HIGH blood sugar include all of the following except:**
    a. Coma
    b. Frequent urination
    c. Fruity smelling breath and urine
    d. Headache

5. **Prior to going for a multi-pitch climb in a national park, a member of your party states she has a severe allergy to bee stings. Your advice to her should be:**
    a. Just bring some diphenhydramine with us in case you get stung
    b. No problem, there won't be any bees
    c. We should cancel the trip
    d. You should get an epinephrine auto-injector from your doctor before we go

ANSWERS
1. c 2. c 3. c 4. a 5. d

CHAPTER 11

Wilderness Wound Management

Objectives:
- Understand the importance of identifying and thoroughly visualizing wounds in the wilderness
- Describe methods to stop bleeding in a step-wise fashion
- Discuss methods to prevent infection of wounds in the wilderness
- Describe recognition of infected wounds
- Identify wounds that require evacuation from the wilderness

> **Case 11.1**
>
> You are backpacking with a group of friends in the wilderness on a multi-day trek. You come across an individual who has a blood-soaked shirt wrapped around his forearm. He states he was free climbing about six hours earlier and fell. You examine his forearm and note an actively bleeding, four-centimeter laceration.
>
> - How should you examine this wound?
> - What steps should you take to stop the bleeding?
> - What is the most important step to prevent infection?
> - Does he require evacuation? What factors determine the need to evacuate victims with wounds from the backcountry?

Assessing the Wound

Injuries to the skin are one the most common problems encountered in the wilderness. Due to numerous environmental, wilderness, and supply issues, it can be difficult to properly evaluate and treat a simple wound. Furthermore, once a wound has been treated, it can be difficult to keep an injury, even a simple abrasion, clean or covered properly.

There are general guidelines that can be used to manage any wound:
- History
- Examination
- Control active bleeding
- Cleaning
- Debridement
- Definitive wound care

Before examining a wound, a history of the injury should be obtained.
- When did the injury occur?
- What caused the wound? Was the penetrating object clean or dirty?
- Has the wound been cleaned in any way?
- Is there any chance that a foreign object (e.g., gravel, a piece of tree branch, etc.) could still be inside the wound? Does it feel like a foreign object is in the wound?
- For wounds to the arms and legs: is there any numbness, loss of peripheral pulse, inability to move fingers/toes, or color changes beyond where the injury appears?

All wounds should be thoroughly examined with a focus on the following areas:
- Type of wound (abrasion, laceration, etc.)
- Location
- Dimensions (width, length, and depth)
- Presence or absence of foreign object (dirt, rocks, teeth, etc.)

Other important principles to consider when examining wounds:
- Ensure the entire wound is visible, even if this requires removing or cutting clothing.
- If the injury is to an extremity, do the following:
  - Ensure that the victim is able to move all joints beyond the wound through a complete range of motion with normal strength.
  - Evaluate the victim's circulation by squeezing the tip of the victim's fingers or toes with one finger over the nail and another over the pad of the finger, for one second. After releasing, the color should return to the nail bed within two to three seconds. If not, the circulation may be compromised. This test is unreliable in cold weather.
- Proper light for examination is paramount. A headlamp is an excellent hands-free tool to improve visualization in the wilderness.

Types of Skin Wounds

Abrasions

- These "road rash" injuries can range from minor scrapes that involve the superficial layers of the skin to injuries that cause major skin disruption, as seen in high-speed crashes.
- More serious injuries may involve muscle tissue and can be serious enough to require skin grafting.
- Most abrasions result in minimal blood loss but can be very painful due to exposure of many nerve endings.
- These injuries are commonly contaminated and contain foreign objects, such as dirt and rocks, depending on how they occurred.

Lacerations

- A cut to the skin is called a laceration
- There are many different types of lacerations:
  - The laceration may be straight, curved, or even star-shaped ("burst").
  - Puncture wounds are lacerations with greater depth than length. These have a higher risk of infection and often have foreign objects embedded deeply in the wound. Due to the depth and unknown pathway, puncture wounds are more difficult to examine and clean.
  - Bites from animals and humans may cause puncture or laceration wounds. Because mouths are full of bacteria, these wounds are at high risk for infection.

Blisters

- Blisters that develop in the wilderness most commonly form due to frictional forces while hiking. Improperly broken-in or poorly fitting shoes are the most common causes.
- A blister is typically preceded by a "hot spot," which is a painful red area formed from the frictional forces. Presentation may range from minor and even painless fluid collections to debilitating injuries that may require evacuation. Infection is the worst complication, although pain and disability are more common.

Burns

- There are two important criteria to be considered with burns:
  - The degree (depth) of the burn
  - The size of the burn in relation to the victim's total body area

Superficial (First Degree) Burn
- The skin is typically reddened, and the victim will likely complain of pain.
- A common example of a superficial burn is sunburn.
- While superficial burns are painful, they are the easiest type of burn to treat and evacuation is generally unnecessary.

Partial Thickness (Second Degree) Burn
- The skin will be blistered and either red or possibly pale white to yellow.
- Partial thickness burns are painful and involve deeper skin damage.
- Partial thickness burns can be significant, especially if they involve a large area of skin.
- Evacuation may be required depending on the extent of the skin (amount of body surface area) involved and the location of the burn.

Full Thickness (Third Degree) Burn
- All layers of the skin have been burned, including blood vessels and nerves in the subcutaneous tissue.
- The flesh may be charred, but the victim generally feels no pain from a full-thickness burn because the nerve endings have been destroyed.
- Painful partial thickness burns may surround the third-degree burn.
- Evacuation is required for any full thickness burn affecting more than 1% TBSA, or if the full thickness burn affects the hands, feet, face, or genitals.

Burn Size
- Burn area should be estimated to help determine the need for evacuation. This can easily be accomplished by using the rule of nines to determine total body surface area (TBSA):

Each arm:	9% TBSA
Each leg:	9% TBSA
Front of trunk:	18% TBSA
Back of trunk:	18% TBSA
Head and neck:	9% TBSA
Groin:	1% TBSA

- Another estimation guide is to use the patient's palm, which represents approximately 1% TBSA.

Treatment of Skin Wounds

Control Active Bleeding

First Step: Direct Pressure

- The first method of control is to apply direct pressure on the wound.
- When applying direct pressure, remember to follow these rules:
  - Use gloves and sterile dressing (if available) to reduce the chance of infection.
  - Apply pressure with the heel of hand directly onto wound for 10-20 minutes.
  - Raise the wound above the level of the heart, if possible
  - Be patient
- Certain wounds are particularly hard to control.
  - Large wounds: because of the large number of blood vessels involved and it is harder to put pressure on the entire wound
  - Scalp wounds: because the scalp has a lot of blood vessels

Second Step: Pressure Dressing +/- Hemostatic Dressing

- A pressure bandage should be applied if there is continued bleeding or if you need your hands to provide other care to the patient.
- How to apply a pressure dressing:
  - Wrap and hold the dressing in place with an elastic bandage (Ace® wrap) or tape that is wrapped circumferentially around the extremity.
  - If you have a special "hemostatic" dressing which is specifically designed to stop bleeding then you should apply this directly to the wound and then wrap it with a pressure dressing.
- If the patient continues to bleed through the pressure dressing:
  - Remove the elastic bandage and place additional dressing on top of the dressing that is already on the wound.
  - Do not remove that initial dressing.
  - Wrap this additional dressing with an elastic bandage.
  - Apply direct pressure with your hand on top of this pressure dressing.
- After applying a pressure bandage, be sure to check distal function and pulse often.

Third Step: Using a Tourniquet

- A tourniquet is a band applied around an arm or leg so tightly that all circulation below the band is cut off.
- While widely viewed as a last resort, a tourniquet can be used initially for a short interval of time to determine the best approach of treatment and evacuation. If you decide to use a tourniquet in this fashion, do not leave it for more than five minutes.
- If you have tried the other methods to stop the bleeding and the wound in continuing to bleed through the dressing, then you should consider a tourniquet as a last resort if you are able to place one.
- The placement of the tourniquet does not mandate that the tourniquet stay in place until the patient reaches definitive medical care. The expectation is that that the rescuer will reassess the wound and the bleeding after the patient has been stabilized in the secondary survey and ongoing assessment stage.
    - Tourniquets are to be used only if the wound is on an arm or leg.
    - Be aware that if a tourniquet cuts off the blood supply for a sufficient period of time to cause tissue damage from lack of oxygen supply, everything below the tourniquet may require amputation.
    - To make a tourniquet, take a strip of cloth at least two inches wide. Never use wire, twine, cord, or any other thin material that will cut the skin.
    - Using an overhand knot, tie the material in a half-knot two inches above to the wound, between the wound and the heart.
    - Place a stick or rod on top of that half-knot and complete the knot on top of the stick.
    - Tighten the bandage by turning the stick until the bandage is tight enough to stop the bleeding.
    - Secure the stick so the tourniquet won't come loose. This may require taping it down.
    - Write on the victim's forehead the time you applied the tourniquet. This is an obvious note to the health care providers who receive the victim in case you are not able to talk with them directly about the care of that victim.

Irrigation

"High-pressure" irrigation is the most important intervention to prevent infection and to decrease bacterial content for most wounds.

- Irrigate the wound with a forceful stream of disinfected water or saline. This can be created a number of ways:
    o If available, use a syringe to create a high-pressure stream for irrigation.
    o Fill a plastic bag or hydration system with the cleanest fluid available (tap water has been shown to protect against infection as effectively as sterile saline). Poke a small hole in a corner of the bag, and then close the top of the bag to create a seal in order to force a stream of water from the bag.
    o A plastic water bottle with an adjustable top may also be used if a stream can be produced.
- Gently pull apart the wound edges while irrigating. Rinse the wound forcefully with the water, protecting your skin and eyes from fluid splashes. The more fluid used to irrigate the wound, the better. Use at least one liter per wound if water is in sufficient supply.
- Do not forcefully drive water deep into puncture wounds; it can push bacteria and debris further into the surrounding tissue.

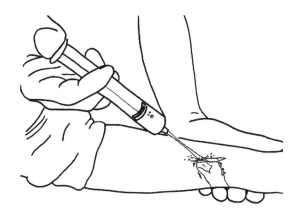

Figure 11.2 Irrigating a Wound

Foreign Matter in Wounds

- It is important to remove visible foreign matter from the wound in order to minimize the chance of infection and to prevent skin tattooing. This may be problematic, particularly if one is unable to adequately visualize the entire wound. Once all visible foreign matter is removed from a wound, another round of irrigation should be performed.

Wound Closure

- The primary goal of wound closure is to bring the wound edges together in order to improve the functional status of the victim and to minimize the scar that results from the wound.
- A common misconception regarding wounds is that closure of the wound decreases the chance of infection. In reality, closure of the wound may increase the chance of infection compared to packing the wound and dressing it properly.
- An important consideration is that there is generally no increase in scarring if one packs and dresses a wound and then closes it three to five days later, as opposed to closing it at the time of injury.
- Packing and dressing a wound with delayed closure is termed *delayed primary closure*. If one is in the wilderness for a period of five days or less, then delayed primary closure is a very good option.

Methods of skin closure that can be utilized in the wilderness that do not involve suturing include the following:

Taping the wound:
- The tape should close the wound so the edges of the wound touch (approximate), but not so tightly that the tape squeezes the wound rigidly shut.
- If needed, cut away the hair around the edges of the wound with scissors so that the tape will adhere better. Do not shave the area around the wound, as shaving may increase the chance of infection.
- Cut the tape into thin strips approximately four to six millimeters in width.
- Place the tape perpendicular to the wound, allowing an adherent length of tape for at least one inch on each side of the wound.
- Place the strips of tape approximately two to five millimeters apart.
- If micropore tape (medical tape) is not available, then one may use duct tape. However, when using the duct tape, punch holes in duct tape from the sticky side out using a safety pin. This allows fluid to drain from the wound through the tape.

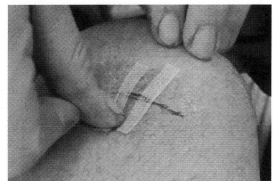

Figure 12.5 Taping a wound - Photo courtesy of Remote Medicine Ireland

Hair-knotting technique to close scalp wounds:
- If the hair is at least one inch long on both sides of the wound, it can be tied or glued together to close the wound edges.
- Separate the hair on each side of the wound.
- On each side of the wound, roll several strands of hair together.
- Pull these strands across the wound to the opposite side. Depending upon the length of the rolled strands, these can be tied or twisted to pull the wound edges together. If the hair is twisted together, applying "super glue" so that the hair does not untwist will hold it more securely.
- Several groups of rolled strands may be needed to close a long wound.

Dressing

Wound dressing is important for protection from the environment and prevention of infection. This may be accomplished in a number of ways:

- If available, apply antibiotic/antiseptic ointment and cover with a sterile, non-stick dressing. Cover this with an absorbent gauze dressing and secure with tape.
- If a commercial non-stick pad or dressing is not available, improvise using a gauze pad and antibiotic/antiseptic ointment. Cover this dressing with an absorbent gauze dressing, then secure with tape.
- If the injury is on a flexible part of the body – an elbow or a finger, for example – immobilize the joint with a splint to prevent reopening of the wound.
- Dressing changes and wound checks should be performed at least once daily in the wilderness. Most infections begin within 48 hours, but aggressive and gas-forming infections may begin within hours.

Topical Antibiotics/Antiseptics

Topical antibiotic/antiseptic ointments are appropriate for all skin wounds.

- Ointments can be obtained over the counter. There is no best ointment, although allergic reactions may be more common if neomycin is a component.

Types of Wounds

Abrasions

- Abrasions should be irrigated as described above.
- In addition to irrigation, abrasions that are very dirty may require vigorous scrubbing in order to remove the embedded dirt and other foreign material.
- Although scrubbing is painful, it is important to ensure proper healing with minimization of infection and tattooing from retained foreign matter.
- Dress and treat as indicated above.

Amputations

- Partial amputations should have the bleeding controlled and then wrapped and evacuated.
- Full amputations
  - Control the bleeding using previously described methods.
  - The amputated part should ideally be wrapped in water-soaked, sterile gauze and then placed in a bag. The bag is then transported on ice with the victim to definitive care as soon as possible.
  - Do not place the amputated part directly on the ice, as this could cause a freezing injury.

Lacerations

Most lacerations can be treated as described in "Treatment of Skin Wounds" above.

Scalp Lacerations
- The extent and severity of scalp lacerations are often initially obscured by surrounding hair that is matted with blood.
- Copious irrigation is often necessary to visualize the laceration.
- Hair may be trimmed if necessary, but this should be limited to the immediate area of the laceration, since the surrounding hair can later be twisted into strands and used to approximate the wound edges.

Facial Lacerations
- Superficial lacerations to the face may be managed in the wilderness.
- Those involving the eyelids or the ears or those with deep injuries require evacuation.
- As with other lacerations, high-pressure irrigation is the method of choice for mechanical cleaning.

Deep Lacerations to the Arm, Hand, or Foot
- Management of deep extremity lacerations in the wilderness requires careful judgment because of the potential involvement of underlying structures.
- This is especially true with the hand, where critical structures lie perilously close to the surface.
- Therefore, a detailed evaluation of all wounds to the arms, hands, and feet should be performed, including these steps:
  - Test the strength of the extremity beyond the wound because tendon injuries may not be obvious at initial evaluation.
  - Evaluate the base of the wound through full range of motion of the extremity because tendon lacerations may easily be missed if examined in just one position.
  - Check sensation beyond the wound. This is easily accomplished by asking the victim to compare sensation beyond the wound with sensation at the same location on the uninvolved arm, hand, leg, or foot.
- Any loss of movement, circulation, or sensation beyond a wound mandates evacuation.

Puncture Wounds

- Puncture wounds should NOT be forcefully irrigated because this may further push in bacteria, dirt and debris.
- Instead, the surface should be thoroughly scrubbed, and the wound should be dressed as indicated above, without closure.
- Puncture wounds should be reevaluated more frequently than simple lacerations, as they are at higher risk for infection.

Bites

- Bites should be cleaned extensively, examined closely for foreign objects, such as teeth, and dressed as described.
- Bites are at higher risk for infection due to bacterial contamination from mouth germs and therefore should be checked regularly.

Blisters

- If a small blister or hot spot forms, protect the area by cutting a hole the size of the blister in a piece of moleskin.
    - Secure the moleskin around the blister to act as a shield to the area.
    - Anchor the moleskin with benzoin or a similar product, and secure with tape.
    - Build up several layers of moleskin or mole foam if necessary. Do not open or puncture small blisters.
- Studies have shown the effectiveness of dual layer blist-o-ban in preventing and treating blisters.
- If the blister is large (2 cm or larger) or ruptured, wash the area and puncture the base of the blister with a sterile needle or safety pin. Carefully remove the external flap of skin from the blister, and apply an antibiotic/antiseptic ointment, covering the blister with a sterile dressing. This can be protected with moleskin or mole foam.
- Inspect daily for signs of infection. If an intact blister appears infected, drain it by removing the external flap and seek medical attention.

Burns

Superficial Burns (First-Degree Burns)
- Treat first-degree burns with aloe-vera gel.
- For comfort, cool the area with damp wet cloths.

Partial-Thickness and Full-Thickness Burns
- Gently clean the burn with cool water and remove loose skin and debris.
- Trim away all loose skin with scissors.
- Blisters larger than 2 cm, those that are leaking, or those that will obviously burst because of rough handling, may be drained and the flap removed carefully.
- Apply a thin layer of Silvadene or other antimicrobial ointment to the burn and cover with a non-adhering, sterile dressing. Change the dressing at least twice daily.
- Do not apply ice to burns for more than 15 minutes, as this will cause more damage due to a potential frostbite injury.

Signs of Infection

These symptoms indicate that the skin is infected:
- Pain that is worse than it was at the time of the initial insult
- Redness around the wound edges that is spreading out from the wound (commonly, there is mild redness/pinkness right at the wound edge)

- Red streaking away from the wound, particularly towards the heart
- Swelling of the wound and the surrounding area
- Pus draining from the wound
- Fever

Evacuation Guidlines

Victims who have wounds with the following characteristics should be considered for evacuation:
- Complex or mutilating wounds
- Grossly contaminated with penetrating debris
- Lacerations of the ear, eyelid, or cartilage
- Penetration of bone, joint, or tendon
- Bites of the hands, legs, or feet
- Amputations

Wounds with signs of infection should be evacuated as soon as possible.

Burn evacuation guidelines include:
- Partial-thickness burns greater than 10% body surface area
- Full-thickness burns greater than 1% body surface area
- Partial- or full-thickness burns involving the face, hands, feet, or genitals
- Electrical burns
- If the burn victim is medically ill
- Burns complicated by smoke or heat inhalation (evidence of smoke inhalation include difficulty breathing, hoarse voice, singed nasal hairs, or carbon in patient's sputum)

Questions

1. **What is the most important intervention to help prevent infection of a wound?**
    a. Antibiotic/antiseptic ointment
    b. High-pressure irrigation
    c. A sterile wound dressing
    d. Removal of very small foreign objects from the wound

2. **Which burn does NOT require evacuation?**
    a. A camper wakes up when his tent has caught on fire because he did not properly put out his campfire. He is able to evacuate from the tent, but is coughing frequently, complains of shortness of breath, and has singed nose hairs.
    b. A victim with burns on the forearm after attempting to treat a snakebite by placing jumper cables adjacent to the area and starting his car.
    c. A victim with four centimeters of redness on the back of the forearm after brushing against hot firewood.
    d. A victim with burns and blistering to the bottom of his foot after stepping on hot coals.

3. **Which of the following is necessary to evaluate when examining a wound in the wilderness?**
    a. Location, extent, and depth of the wound
    b. Presence or absence of dirt, debris, or foreign objects
    c. Sensation and circulation beyond the wound
    d. All of the above

4. **Which wound requires evacuation?**
    a. A two cm laceration of the head secured by tying strands of hair together
    b. A puncture wound of the foot that has developed surrounding redness, has pus draining from it, and is extremely painful upon which to walk
    c. A three-day-old two cm arm laceration that has some redness around it without pus or worsening pain
    d. A four cm leg laceration that has been irrigated, has no foreign body, bone, tendon, or joint involvement, and is secured with tape

5. **Which is the best way to treat a simple friction blister the size of a dime?**
    a. Clean the area, place a ring of moleskin over it, and cover it with athletic tape
    b. Ignore it; most blisters rupture or stop hurting sooner or later
    c. Puncture with a needle, remove the flap, and cover with athletic tape
    d. Place a ring of moleskin over the blister, cover everything with tape, and evacuate the victim for antibiotics

6. **For which of the following wounds should the use of a tourniquet be considered?**
    a. An amputation of half of the little finger
    b. A partial amputation of the leg at the level of the knee, sustained in a high-speed four-wheeler collision, with bleeding controlled by direct pressure and compression bandages
    c. A rapidly bleeding scalp laceration that continues despite 30 minutes of pressure
    d. An artery laceration at the elbow due to an open fracture from a 15-foot fall that continues to bleed despite 30 minutes of direct pressure and compression bandages

7. **What is the best way to transport amputated digits?**
    a. In milk
    b. In the victim's pocket
    c. Wrapped in sterile water-soaked gauze, placed in a bag and transported on ice
    d. Placed directly on ice and then placed in a plastic bag

8. **Which best describes a partial-thickness burn?**
    a. A large burn with exposed muscle and bone
    b. A painful area of redness without blistering or tissue loss
    c. A painful area of redness with blistering
    d. A burn that has a central painless white area

ANSWERS
1. b   2. c   3. d   4. b   5. a   6. d   7. d   8. c

CHAPTER 12

Heat-Induced Injuries

Objectives:
- Be able to list factors that make someone susceptible to heat illness
- Be able to describe the etiology and management of victims with heat cramps and heat syncope
- Know the similarities and differences between heat exhaustion and heat stroke
- Discuss methods to help prevent heat-related illness
- Know methods of cooling, which method(s) is best in heat illness, and when to stop active cooling
- Be able to list evacuation guidelines for victims with heat illness

> # Case 12.1
>
> During a long distance running event, three victims are brought to your first aid station:
>
> Victim #1: A 27-year-old female "passed out" while standing at a hydration table, where she had stopped to drink some fluids. She wakes shortly after falling to the ground. She is alert and oriented to person, place, time, and event. She denies dizziness, nausea, or weakness and asks if she can continue running.
>
> Victim #2: A 42-year-old male complains of severe spasms in his right calf muscle. He has been drinking large amounts of pure water throughout the day.
>
> Victim #3: A 35-year-old is brought to the aid station by bystanders. They state that the victim was moving erratically and "just not acting right." The victim is obviously confused about the situation. He is covered with sweat and is agitated and warm to the touch.
>
> - What type of heat illness does each victim have?
> - How should each victim be managed?
> - Can any of these victims continue the race?
> - Who needs to be evacuated immediately?

Dehydration

- Dehydration occurs when more water and fluids are exiting the body than are entering the body.
- 75% of the body is made up of water found inside cells, within blood vessels, and between cells.
- Survival in the wilderness requires a rather sophisticated water management system.
- Thirst indicates when a person needs to increase fluid intake.
- Although water is lost constantly throughout the day as we breathe, sweat, urinate, and defecate, we can replenish the water in our body by drinking fluids.
- The body can also shift water around to areas where it is more needed if dehydration begins to occur.
- The immediate causes of dehydration include not enough water, too much water loss or some combination of the two.
- Additional causes of dehydration include:
  - Diarrhea
  - Vomiting
  - Sweating
  - Diabetes
  - Higher altitude

Symptoms of Dehydration

- The first symptoms of dehydration include headache, thirst, darker urine and decreased urine production.
- Urine color is one of the best indicators of a person's hydration level - clear urine means you are well hydrated and darker urine means you are dehydrated.
- As the condition progresses to moderate dehydration, symptoms include:
  - Dry mouth
  - Lethargy
  - Muscle weakness
  - Dizziness

- Severe dehydration is characterized by extreme versions of symptoms mentioned above as well as:
  - Lack of sweating
  - Sunken eyes
  - Low blood pressure
  - Increased heart beat
  - Fever
  - Delirium
  - Unconsciousness

Treatment of Dehydration

- Replenishing the fluid level in the body.
- Consuming clear fluids such as water, clear broths, frozen water or sports drinks.
- People who are dehydrated should avoid drinks containing caffeine such as coffee, tea, and sodas.
- Prevention is really the most important treatment for dehydration.
- Consuming plenty of fluids and foods that have high water content (such as fruits and vegetables) is essential to prevent dehydration.

Heat and the Body

- The body produces heat in two ways: the basic metabolic rate (BMR) and exercise metabolism.
- The body regulates temperature like a furnace. It is constantly producing heat and then dispersing it through various processes.
- Heat can be lost through four processes: conduction, convection, radiation, and evaporation
  - Conduction is the process of losing heat through physical contact with another object or body. For example, if you were to sit on a metal chair, the heat from your body would transfer to the cold metal chair.
  - Convection is the process of losing heat through the movement of air or water molecules across the skin. The use of a fan to cool off the body is one example of convection. The amount of heat loss from convection is dependent upon the airflow or in aquatic exercise, the water flow over the skin. This is where the wind-chill factor takes place.
  - Radiation is a form of heat loss through infrared rays. This involves the transfer of heat from one object to another, with no physical contact involved. For example, the sun transfers heat to the earth through radiation.
  - Evaporation is the process of losing heat through the conversion of water to gas (evaporation of sweat). It utilizes convection, conduction and radiation. In order for evaporation to work, sweat on the skin must evaporate and not drip off the skin.
- If the ability to remove heat from the body is lost, then the body temperature will rise and heat illnesses will occur.

Risk Factors for Heat Illness

Medical Conditions

- Heart disease
- Dehydration
- Vomiting
- Diarrhea
- Fever
- Previous heat exhaustion or heat stroke

Environmental Conditions

- Exercise in a hot climate, particularly if there is high humidity
- Inappropriate clothing (occlusive, heavy, or vapor-impermeable)
- Lack of acclimatization
- Decreased fluid intake
- Hot environments (inside of tents or autos in the sun, hot tubs, saunas)

Drugs & Toxins

- Alcohol
- Antihistamines (including diphenhydramine <Benadryl>)
- Certain motion sickness medications, such as meclizine and dramamine
- Cocaine, amphetamines, and other stimulant drugs

Other Risk Factors

- Salt and/or water depletion
- Obesity

Types of Heat Illness

Heat Cramps

Heat cramps occur when significant salt and water losses are replaced with solutions not containing sufficient salt (sodium chloride or NaCl). Inadequate salt repletion can eventually lead to involuntary contraction of skeletal muscles (cramp). Common characteristics of heat cramps include the following:
- Brief, intermittent, involuntary contractions of skeletal muscles
- Most commonly involve the calves, but may occur in any muscle
- Usually only occur in a single muscle or muscle group and are quite painful
- The victim with heat cramps will classically give a history of the following:
  - Prolonged activity in a hot environment
  - Attempted hydration, typically with a non-electrolyte containing solution, such as plain water
  - Poor salt/electrolyte intake

Treatment
- Mild cases
  - Oral salt replacement.
  - This can be easily made with ¼ to ½ teaspoon of table salt added to a quart of water.
- Severe cases
  - If not responding to the above treatment, the individual may require intravenous fluids and should be evacuated.

Heat Syncope

Syncope is the medical term for "passing out," usually a brief loss of consciousness. Heat syncope typically occurs when a dehydrated individual stands in a hot environment for an extended period of time. When a person stands, blood pools in the legs, decreasing the amount of blood that returns to the heart. This, in combination with dehydration and dilated blood vessels from the hot environment, can decrease blood flow to the brain and cause the individual to faint. Prior to actually losing consciousness, the victim may have the following signs and symptoms:
- Lightheadedness
- Vertigo / dizziness
- Dimming or graying of vision
- Restlessness
- Nausea
- Yawning

These symptoms and the actual loss of consciousness usually resolve once the victim is lying flat, as this facilitates redistribution of blood from the legs back to the brain.

Treatment
- The loss of consciousness should be brief, on the order of several seconds up to two minutes.
- Treatment to improve blood flow to the brain should be instituted
    - Lay the victim flat on their back (supine)
    - Elevate the feet to improve venous return back to the heart
    - Loosen tight or constrictive clothing
    - Remove from direct sunlight
    - Move to a cool area if possible
    - Have the victim drink fluids once consciousness is regained
- Assess the victim for other injuries that may have resulted from the fall

Heat Exhaustion

Heat exhaustion is a form of heat illness that results from a significant heat stress. Heat exhaustion is part of a continuum of heat illnesses that progress to heat stroke.

Symptoms
- Weakness
- Lightheadedness
- Fatigue
- Nausea with or without vomiting
- Headache
- Thirst
- Rapid heartbeat and breathing
- Profuse sweating

Treatment
- Stop all physical activity.
- Replace fluids and electrolytes liberally. With heat exhaustion, oral hydration as discussed below is appropriate.
- Remove the victim from direct sunlight into a cool, shaded area.
- Loosen restrictive clothing.
- If the victim is hyperthermic (core body temperature is > 38 °C or 100.4 °F), take active cooling measures. In the wilderness, there are limited resources to actively cool a victim.
- The best way to cool a hyperthermic victim is through **evaporative cooling**.
    - Remove most of the victim's clothing and make them "sopping wet" with tepid (room temperature) water. While it may seem paradoxical to cool a hyperthermic victim with warm water, the warm temperature of the water helps to prevent shivering and keeps the skin blood vessels dilated, which allows for heat exchange. Cold water might lead to shivering and constriction of the blood vessels in the skin. However, if only cold water is available, use it.
    - Fan the victim with anything that will increase air movement across the skin. This air flow will result in evaporation of water from the skin, which cools the victim.
    - Shivering will increase core body temperature and should be avoided.
- Oral hydration should adhere to the following guidelines:
    - Cool/cold water or sports drink
    - Beverage should not exceed 6% carbohydrate content. Increased carbohydrate content inhibits fluid absorption. You can dilute most sports drinks with water to achieve a better concentration.
    - A general rule is that every pound lost to sweat should be replenished with 500 mL or two cups of fluid.
    - The treatment goal for mild heat exhaustion should be 1 to 2 liters of oral fluids over two to four hours.

Heat Stroke

- Heat stroke is a true medical emergency that is classically defined by the following:
  - Severe hyperthermia (core temperature > 40°C or 104°F)
  - Central nervous system (CNS) disturbances such as alteration in the level of consciousness, confusion, or seizures
  - Lack of active sweating
- However, experience has shown that waiting for the appearance of these three symptoms is too strict and may delay critical treatment.
- Any person who has any of the following symptoms in a hot environment should be treated as having heat stroke:
  - Unsteady gait (often one of the first manifestations of heat stroke)
  - Irritability
  - Confusion
  - Combativeness
  - Bizarre behavior
  - Seizures
  - Hallucinations
  - Coma (very late finding)
- Diminished or lack of sweating is classically associated with heat stroke; however, it is typically a late finding and cannot be relied upon to make an accurate diagnosis. Typically, heat stroke victims will be covered in sweat until very late stages of the illness.
- The key to treatment and prevention of heat stroke is in the understanding that heat exhaustion and heat stroke are not separate entities, but are a continuum of the same illness. The onset of any alteration in mental status should alert the wilderness medicine provider that a victim is suffering from significant heat illness.

Treatment
- The primary goal of treatment for heat stroke is to facilitate rapid cooling, which can be accomplished by evaporative cooling as discussed previously.
- Additionally, one may place ice packs or cold compresses in areas where large blood vessels are superficial, such as the neck, axilla, groin, and scalp.
- Most persons will not have a rectal thermometer to measure temperature. However, it may be used when one is available:
  - The goal of treatment is to drop the temperature to below 40°C (104°F) as rapidly as possible.
  - Active cooling efforts should be discontinued around 39°C (102.2°F) to avoid overshoot to a condition of hypothermia, which can occur with very successful cooling efforts.

Prevention

Hydration

- Drink at least four to eight ounces of water or sports drink every 15-20 minutes during mild to moderate physical activity, depending on the ambient environmental temperature and humidity.
- Hydrate with a goal of clear urine instead of a fixed amount of intake.
- Consume salt-containing foods or add salt to water if exposed to heat for time periods greater than two to three hours, especially if using only water for hydration.
- To make a salt solution, add one-fourth to one-half teaspoon of table salt to a liter of fluid. Flavored drinks that are cold are more palatable.
- Most commercially available sports drinks should be diluted with an equal amount of water for ideal electrolyte concentration.

Heat Dissipation

- Wear loose-fitting clothing that will allow for air circulation and increased evaporation.
- Avoid direct sunlight when possible and wear light-colored clothing.
- Douse with cool fluids or cool misting spray frequently.

Heat Acclimatization

Heat acclimatization decreases the incidence of heat injuries and improves performance in hot environments. The general guidelines for acclimatization include the following:

- Adults should gradually increase the time and intensity of activity in a hot environment over 7 to 10 days.
- Children and elderly people require 10 to 14 days to maximize acclimatization.
- Those who are from temperate or cold climates and will be traveling into a hot environment can acclimatize by going into a sauna or steam room for increasing amounts of time each day, beginning 7 to 10 days before making the trip.
- De-acclimatization usually occurs within one to two weeks of being removed from the hot environment. In such a situation, acclimatization must be repeated if necessary.

Evacuation Guidelines

- A victim who suffers a fainting episode thought to be heat-related should only have brief loss of consciousness and recover quickly. Any victim who endures a prolonged loss of consciousness, persistent pre-syncope signs and symptoms upon awakening, more than one episode of passing out, or signs of heat stroke should be evacuated.
- A victim with severe heat cramps that do not respond to oral salt solutions, or a victim who suffers diffuse and multiple cramps should also be considered for evacuation, depending on the situation.
- Heat exhaustion victims *may not* need to be evacuated:
  - As long as the victim can adequately be protected from the environment.
  - In mild cases, close observation in the field for development of heat stroke, as well as cessation of activities for 24-48 hours, is recommended.
  - If the victim develops behavioral changes, records a temperature above 39°C (102.2°F), or has a fainting episode while under observation, he should be considered a potential heat stroke victim and be evacuated immediately.
- Heat stroke is a serious medical emergency, so any victim with signs or symptoms of heat stroke should be evacuated as soon as possible.

Questions

1. **All of the following increase the risk of heat illness except:**
   a. History of heat injury
   b. Diarrhea
   c. Alcohol
   d. All of the above increase the risk of heat injury

2. **Heat cramps are most likely to occur in which victim?**
   a. A runner on a hot day drinking water alternated with a sports drink
   b. A runner on a hot day not rehydrating with anything
   c. A runner on a hot day drinking 1 liter of only water per hour for several hours
   d. A runner on a hot day drinking 1 liter of only water per hour for two hours

3. **Which one of the following is the most important difference between heat stroke and heat exhaustion?**
   a. Altered mental status
   b. Core body temperature
   c. The presence or absence of sweating
   d. The presence of vomiting

4. **Which one of the following is the most effective way to cool a victim under most conditions?**
   a. Cold water immersion
   b. Cold water evaporative cooling
   c. Ice packs to the axilla/groin
   d. Tepid water evaporative cooling

5. **Acclimatization to a hot environment should take how long for the average adult?**
   a. 1-3 days
   b. 4-6 days
   c. 7-10 days
   d. 11-14 days

ANSWERS
1. d   2. c   3. a   4. d   5. c

CHAPTER 13
Hypothermia and Cold Injuries

Objectives:
- Understand the mechanisms by which the body loses and gains heat
- Recognize and diagnose hypothermia, frostbite, and other cold-related injuries
- Understand the principles of backcountry treatment of cold injuries
- Learn about prevention of these conditions when exposed to cold weather

> **Case 13.1**
>
> While on a cold weather backpacking trip, you come upon a solo hiker who became lost and now has been outside much longer than expected. He is shivering uncontrollably and appears to be confused.
>
> - What are the ways that heat is lost from the body?
> - Should he be evacuated?
> - What is the severity of his hypothermia?
> - How should you treat him?

Hypothermia

Mild hypothermia

- Defined as a core body temperature ranging from 32 to 35°C (90.0 to 95°F)
- Signs of mild hypothermia include the following:
  - Pale and cold skin secondary to blood vessel constriction
  - Uncontrollable shivering as the body attempts to produce heat
  - Varying degrees of confusion, unsteady gait, and disorientation
  - Frequent urination
  - Elevated pulse and breathing rate

Moderate hypothermia

- Defined as a core temperature ranging from 28 to 32°C (82.0 to 90.0°F)
- Signs of moderate hypothermia include the following:
  - Decreased rates of blood pressure, pulse, and breathing
  - Severe confusion as well as dilated pupils and muscle rigidity
- Unless rewarming is possible, the patient will eventually cool to ambient temperature and die

Severe hypothermia

- Defined as a core temperature below 28°C (82.0°F)
- Signs of severe hypothermia include the following:
  - Deep coma with dilated pupils and muscular rigidity
  - Pulse may be as low as 10-20 beats per minute and may be difficult to feel
  - People in severe hypothermia often appear to be dead

Treatment

- The most important consideration in treating hypothermia is removing the patient from the situation that caused them to become hypothermic.
- If a patient cannot be evacuated, attempts should be made to get him or her to a shelter that is out of cold, wet, and windy conditions that may precipitate further heat loss.
- Wet clothes should be removed, and patients should be wrapped in dry blankets, if possible.
- Anything that can be done to help rewarm the patient will be helpful, such as sitting them by a fire or giving them warm liquids. It is important however to avoid beverages such as alcohol or heavily caffeinated drinks, which may worsen hypothermia.

- In a rescue situation, it is important to remember the premise that "no one is dead until they are warm and dead." People suffering from severe hypothermia may be severely comatose, though alive, and may recover with proper medical care.

The following are specific recommendations for treatment of the different levels of hypothermia in the field. However, keep in mind that field treatment of hypothermia is notoriously difficult, and arrangements should begin for evacuation as soon as it is determined that the patient cannot actively rewarm himself or herself:

Mild hypothermia
- Remove the patient from the elements and move into shelter to avoid further heat loss.
- If the person is wet, undress them and dress them in dry clothes and wrap them in blankets taking special care to cover the head and neck to avoid heat loss.
- Warmed, sweetened beverages may be helpful.
- Limited exercise may generate some heat (this is not advised in moderate and severe hypothermia).

Moderate hypothermia (in addition to the treatments mentioned above)
Apply *mild* heat to the head, neck, chest, armpits, and groin of the patient using hot water bottles, wrapped commercial heating pads, or warm moist towels.
- These patients should be evacuated

Severe hypothermia
- It is important to consider that patients suffering from this condition may exhibit altered mental status if they are still conscious. Therefore, it is vital to ignore pleas of "Leave me alone, I'm okay" because these individuals are in serious trouble.
- Inhalation of warm, humidified air into the lungs can aid in rewarming key areas of the body such as the head, neck, and thorax.
- Care must be taken in handling patients suffering from this condition as extremely cold core temperatures can cause irritability of the heart muscle. Even a small bump can cause the heart to fibrillate and stop beating effectively.
- Above all else, it is crucial to closely monitor individuals suffering from this condition. Remember that severe hypothermia may mimic other medical conditions and may mimic death as well.

Prevention

- The single most important aspect in hypothermia prevention is adequate preparation.
    - Maintain awareness of weather conditions
    - Bring the proper gear
    - Design a contingency plan in case the worst should occur
    - Remember also that the weather does not need to be sub-zero in order for hypothermia to set in

- Should the unexpected occur and you are faced with this situation, the following is a list of things that can be done to help prevent hypothermia:
    - Find or create a shelter
    - Cover exposed areas of the body
    - Wear several loosely fitting layers of clothing
    - Conserve, share, and create warmth
    - Increase heat production through voluntary muscle movement
    - Consume warm beverages and food
    - Monitor for signs and symptoms of hypothermia.

Frostbite

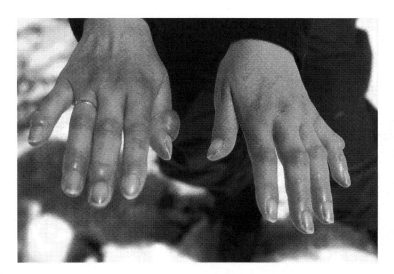

Figure 13.1 Frostbitten Hands

- Frostbite is the freezing (ice crystal formation) of skin that may involve deeper tissues
- Frostbite is divided into four degrees and is based on the depth of tissue damage in a manner similar to burns.
- First and second degree frostbite are considered to be superficial and typically heal well with minor long-term consequences, while third and fourth degree frostbite are deeper and associated with very significant permanent damage and tissue loss.
- The following are descriptions of the different degrees of frostbite:

First Degree (Superficial)

- This involves the superficial layers of skin
- The skin appears pale and white while frozen and is numb to the touch
- During rewarming, there will be pain and redness of the involved area
- After rewarming, the area will be swollen and continue to be red for a period of hours

Second Degree (Superficial)

- This involves deeper layers of the skin
- The skin appears pale and white while frozen and is numb to the touch
- During rewarming, there will be pain and redness of the involved area
- After rewarming, the area will be swollen and continue to be red for a period of hours
- In addition to the redness, the skin will develop blisters over the area of involvement. These blisters will be filled with a clear fluid.

Third Degree (Deep)

- This involves complete freezing of the skin and tissue layers under the skin.
- The skin appears pale and white while frozen and is numb to the touch.
- During rewarming, there will be pain, redness and swelling of the involved area.
- After rewarming, the area will be swollen and continue to be red for a period of hours to days.
- In addition to the redness, the skin will develop blisters over the area of involvement. These blisters will be filled with a bloody fluid.

Fourth Degree (Deep)

- This involves the skin and much deeper tissues including muscle, tendon, and bone.
- The area of involvement appears pale and white while frozen.
- Numb to the touch, the skin has a "chunk of wood" type of consistency.
- During rewarming, there will be significant pain, redness and swelling of the involved area.
- After rewarming, the area will be swollen and continue to be red for a period of hours to days.
- In addition to the redness, the skin will develop blisters over the area of involvement. These blisters will be filled with a bloody fluid.
- Mottled skin with bluish discoloration forms a deep, dry, black crusted lesion.

Treatment

- In general, all frostbite should be treated in a medical facility by health care providers.
  - Thawing of a frozen body part is a very painful process that usually requires narcotic pain medications and other medications such as antibiotics and anti-inflammatory agents.
  - An inappropriate or inadequate thawing process will cause the patient more harm.
- Prior to rewarming, treat the patient with ibuprofen 400 mg, if they have no allergy to it.
- The primary treatment is rapid rewarming in a controlled manner.
  - This should only occur when there is no chance of the person refreezing the area of involvement.
    - Refreezing of a previously thawed frostbitten body part will result in a significant increase in the amount of damage that occurs.
    - A failure to rewarm in a rapid manner will increase tissue damage.
- The optimal method of rewarming is to place the affected body part into gently circulated water that has been warmed to 40-42°C (104-108°F).
  - This should be done for at least 15-30 minutes or until skin regains pliability and returns to its normal color.
  - A good rule of thumb is to heat the water until it approximates the temperature of a hot tub.
  - The temperature must be closely monitored with a thermometer. If it is too hot, it will burn the skin, which will worsen the injury. If it is too cool, it will delay thawing, which will worsen the injury.
- Additional measures that may be taken in the wilderness setting include the following:
  - Remove all wet clothing and replace it with dry clothes.
  - Remove any tight or constrictive clothing.
  - If possible, wrap the involved area with clean gauze. If the frostbite involves the hands or feet, separate the fingers toes with dry gauze in addition to wrapping the hand/foot.
  - Elevate the extremity to reduce swelling.
  - Pad the skin with cotton or gauze.
  - Treat pain with medicines such as acetaminophen and ibuprofen.
- DO-NOTS OF FROSTBITE TREATMENT
  - Do not attempt thawing by heating with dry heat such as a fire. The fact that the temperature is not controlled may lead to delay in thawing but may also burn the area as the area is numb.
  - Do not thaw the area if there is any chance that the area will refreeze. If a body part undergoes freezing again soon after being rewarmed the extent of the injury is much worse than if there was just a delay in the thawing. An example is the person with the frostbitten foot in the wilderness. It is better to have that person walk out on the frozen foot than to risk a refreezing injury, if it is possible.
  - Do not rub the area when it is frozen or thawing as that will worsen the injury.
  - Do not rub the area with snow. This is an old recommendation that was proven to be harmful in the 1950s.

Prevention

- Covering susceptible areas of skin with properly fitting dry clothing and footgear is essential during prolonged exposure to cold weather. To this end, a waterproof bag containing an extra pair of socks and undergarments may come in handy.
- Maintain a good diet and stay well hydrated.
- Consumption of alcohol and smoking cigarettes may also contribute to frostbite and should therefore be avoided.
- In extreme situations, putting one's hand or feet in his or her partner's armpits may provide some added warmth.
- Continuous movement, including frequent contraction and relaxation of extremities, may also be helpful.

Frostnip

- Frostnip is a cold injury to the skin, but the actual tissue does not freeze as with frostbite.
- It is the result of prolonged skin exposure to cold temperatures.
- Frostnip can be a **precursor to frostbite** and should therefore be taken seriously.
- Signs of frostnip include the following:
  - The affected area will be red and swollen, but the skin will stay soft and pliable.
  - Numbness and tingling are possible but should resolve after rewarming.
  - Frostnip only has mild pain when rewarming.
  - Pain and skin cracking are possible in areas that are repeatedly frostnipped, potentially leading to infection.

  Areas that are most commonly affected include fingers, toes, ears, and cheeks.

Treatment

- Rewarm the injured area using water, fire, or another heat source.
- Take care not to rub frostnipped areas as this may promote tissue damage.
- Unlike frostbite, these injuries should always be rewarmed even if still exposed to a cold environment since the tissue has not yet been damaged and will only become damaged if the process is allowed to continue.

Evacuation Guidelines

Hypothermia
- Mild – Evacuation is a judgment call. If the patient can be removed from the elements, can be dressed in dry clothing, and can adequately rewarm himself or herself, evacuation is not absolutely necessary.
- Moderate and Severe – Both definitely require evacuation.

Frostbite
- All frostbite should be evacuated from the field as it is difficult to determine the degree of frostbite until the area is thawed.

Questions

1. **In which degree of hypothermia is uncontrollable shivering a feature?**
    a. Mild hypothermia
    b. Moderate hypothermia
    c. Severe hypothermia

2. **Which one of the following is not a step that should be taken to prevent further hypothermia in the victim who is cold?**
    a. Getting the patient to shelter
    b. Drinking warm beverages
    c. Smoking cigarettes
    d. Removing wet clothing

3. **Which one of the following is an important medication that you must administer to the patient who has frostbite before they undergo rapid rewarming of the frostbitten body part?**
    a. Acetaminophen (Tylenol)
    b. Epinephrine (EpiPen)
    c. Ibuprofen
    d. Nitroglycerin

4. **Which degree of frostbite is associated with full-thickness skin involvement in addition to muscle and tendon involvement with blisters containing red fluid?**
    a. First degree
    b. Second degree
    c. Third degree
    d. Fourth degree

5. **When should frostbite not be treated in the field with rewarming?**
    a. If the patient will be promptly evacuated
    b. If the patient is diabetic
    c. If there is a possibility of refreezing

6. **How does frostnip differ from frostbite?**
    a. There is no ice crystal formation in frostnip
    b. Permanent damage occurs, but it is very minor with frostnip but not first-degree frostbite
    c. Frostnip only involves the surface of the skin and frostbite goes down to the muscle
    d. Frostbite has red, blood containing blisters, whereas frostnip has white to clear blisters

ANSWERS
1. a 2. c 3. c 4. d 5. c 6. a

CHAPTER 14

Bites and Stings

This chapter will train you on general issues related to preventing and treating bites and stings from the following land creatures:

- Domesticated Animals
- Wild Animals
- Snakes
- Mosquitoes
- Spiders
- Ticks
- Hymenoptera
- Scorpions

Case 14.1

You and a friend are camping. You awake to roars and thumps outside your tent. Looking out the tent flap, you see your friend on the ground in the fetal position as a black bear knocks him around. You see potato chips scattered all over the campground.

- What is the best approach to stopping the bear from attacking your friend?
- Would your approach be different if you were in Canada and it was a Grizzly bear?
- How should you treat him?

Case 14.2

You are camping with a friend when he comes running out of the woods being chased by several bees. After he has been running approximately one-fourth of a mile, the bees stop chasing him. Your friend comes to you with approximately 10 stings, several of which still contain the stinger with the sac attached. He does not have any breathing problems. He feels slightly dizzy from the whole event but does not appear sick.

- What is the best way to remove the stingers from the wounds?
- If you have an EpiPen®, should you use it on your friend?
- Does he require evacuation from the site, or can you sit and watch him?

Case 14.3

A 24-year-old female has been swimming in the ocean when she notes the onset of an immediate stinging sensation on her arm and leg. Some 30 feet away you notice what appear to be a number of small "sails" floating on the water. On exam, you notice a rash that has a "tentacle-like" appearance.

- What should the immediate treatment be on the beach?
- What is the cause?
- What are the signs of severe envenomation one can see?

Domesticated Animals

General

- The majority (80% - 90%) of domesticated animal bites are dog bites.
- Cat bites account for 5% - 15% of domestic animal bites.
- Victims of bites are often the pet owners or members of the pet owner's family.

Wilderness Care
- Direct pressure should be used to stop bleeding.
- Wounds that do not break the skin can be treated with ice and pain medications such as acetaminophen and ibuprofen.
- The wound should be irrigated and cleaned as soon as possible, especially if the patient is greater than one hour from definitive medical care.
  - Sterile water is not required, but the cleaner the water the better.
  - Soap in the water increases the efficacy of cleaning and may decrease the potential for rabies.
  - Rinsing the wound (irrigation) should be done under high pressure.
  - Dress the wound with a clean cloth.

Wound Infections
- Infection is common with animal bites.
- Bites are tetanus-prone wounds. Everyone should always ensure that their tetanus immunizations are up-to-date prior to entering the wilderness as skin injuries are very common.

Rabies
- Rabies is more commonly found in bats, raccoons, and skunks than dogs in the United States.
- In most parts of the world, dog bites are the most common source of rabies.
- Good wound cleansing can decrease the risk for rabies infection.
- The Center for Disease Control (CDC) in the United States has a 24-hour helpline that can assist in determining the need to administer the rabies vaccine. www.cdc.gov/rabies

Dog Bites

Prevention
- Never leave a child alone with a dog.
- Do not pet other people's dogs without permission.
- Do not kiss a dog.
- Do not physically separate fighting dogs; instead use a hose.
- Never take a bone or toy away from an unfamiliar dog.
- Never pet or step over a sleeping dog.

Treatment
- Immediate patient management and wound care should be performed as outlined above.
- Wounds should be monitored closely for infection

Cat Bites

Treatment
- Immediate patient management and wound care as outlined above.
- Cat bites have a higher infection rate in comparison to other domestic animals because they are more commonly puncture-type wound.

Wild Animals

General

Prevention
- Animal behavior holds the key to prevention of most animal attacks.
- Aside from large carnivores, most animals do not attack humans unprovoked.
- The most common examples of human provocation of wild animals occur during time of animal capture or restraint.
- Even the shyest animal can inflict a life-threatening injury when cornered.

Bear Attacks

Background
- North American bears include the brown (grizzly and Kodiak), American black, and polar bears. Brown bears vary in color from dark brown to blonde and can be distinguished from black bears due to their prominent shoulder hump and rounded face.
- Bears are fast (up to 40 mph) and large (140 to 1,400 pounds) with keen senses of smell and hearing.
- Bear attacks are more common in the summer months because the bears are not hibernating and there are more visitors in the parks.
- The most common scenario ending in a brown bear attack is a sudden unexpected close encounter.
- The wounds are described as a mauling, but the bear often inflicts the injuries and leaves without inflicting wounds to its maximum potential.
- Situations that are more fatal include encroaching on a bear that is wounded, with a cub, or near a carcass.
- In contrast to the brown bears, black bears rarely attack because of close encounters. Black female bears with cubs are more apt to flee an area if the human shows aggression.

Prevention
- Make noise, such as talking, and allow the bears to move away from you.
- Be cautious in environments where a bear may not be able to hear you such as near loud streams and in uneven terrain.
- Avoid common bear areas such as streams with spawning fish, berry groves, and carcasses.
- Camp in the open and cook your food away from your sleeping area.
- Sleep upriver from your cooking site.
- Maintain a clean camping site. Keep odorous products away from your sleeping gear.
- Find a spot to hang your food at night above the ground where a bear cannot reach it.
- If spotted by a bear, allow it to see you as human by stepping forward to allow the bear a full view of you.
- If able to avoid an attack, retreat by waiting until the bear has left the area and move in the opposite direction.
- Pepper spray may be useful if discharged directly at a charging bear's head when it is within thirty feet. Pepper spray is not to be used as mosquito repellant and pepper spray sprayed in a camp may actually serve as a bear attractant.
- If you encounter a brown bear, take the following actions:
  - Do <u>not</u> look into the bear's eyes, as it is a sign of aggression.
  - Do <u>not</u> make any sudden movements.
  - Do <u>not</u> run.
  - Do <u>not</u> act aggressively towards the bear.
  - Just stand your ground but submissively.
  - If attacked, get into the fetal position with your neck protected as they are "head oriented."

- If you encounter a black bear, take the following actions:
  - Yell, throw things, and act aggressively towards the bear as they usually will flee in response to aggression.
  - If attacked – fight back as a black bear is likely viewing you as food
  - If rolled onto your back, protect your face with your elbows.

Treatment
- The possibility for significant injury is high.
- All bear attack victims should be considered trauma victims and immediately evacuated.

Cougar Attacks

- The North American cougar (mountain lion, puma) has come into contact with humans with increasing frequency.
- Cougars are most commonly encountered in the western United States.
- Cougars hunt by stealth, then pounce and break the victim's neck.
- As with lions, cougars can potentially be scared off by the victim's aggressive behavior towards the animal. This is less likely in the case of a cougar with a cub or a wounded cougar.
- When confronted by a cougar, you should face it, talk very loudly, and make yourself appear as a threat.
- Do not turn and run away from a cougar.
- If you have small children with you, pick them up as the cougar preferentially attacks children.
- If the cougar attacks, fight back using anything including rocks, sticks, bare fists, and fishing poles.

Snakes

General

- North America has two native types of poisonous snakes: the pit viper and the coral snake.
- The overwhelming majority of envenomation in the U.S. come from pit vipers.
- Annually, there are approximately 9,000 snakebites reported in the U.S.
- From 1983 to 1998 there were only 10 deaths attributed to snake envenomation.

Pit Vipers

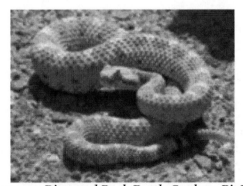

Figure 14.1 Diamond Back Rattle Snake – Pit Viper

Background
- In the United States, pit vipers include the rattlesnake, copper head, and water moccasin (cotton mouth).

- Pit vipers have a specific recognizable anatomy:
  - Triangle shaped heads
  - Catlike pupils
  - Heat sensing pits between eyes and nose
- Venom is dispersed from a tunnel in the fangs.
- Approximately 25% of snakebites are "dry bites." This means that the snake injects no venom.
- Each snake has a varying potency of its venom based on multiple factors:
  - Emotional state of snake
  - Species of snake as well as its size and age
  - Time of year that the bite occurs
  - Location of bite (more dangerous near vital organs)
  - Amount of venom injected (snakes can regulate the amount of venom released)

Clinical manifestations of pit viper envenomation
- Severe burning at the bite site within minutes
- Soft tissue swelling outward from the bite
- Blood oozing from the bite
- Bluish discoloration at the bite site and further down the limb
- Nausea and vomiting
- Weakness
- Rubber, minty, or metallic taste in the mouth
- Numbness of mouth and tongue
- Uncontrollable muscle contractions
- Increased heart and breathing rate
- Difficulty breathing in severe cases
- Shock

Treatment
- Keep the victim calm and evacuate while minimizing physical activity.
- Support the airway, breathing, and circulation while transporting.
- Tight-fitting jewelry and clothing should be removed to avoid a tourniquet effect.
- The swelling edge should be marked every 15 minutes for physicians and the hospital to assess the severity of the envenomation.
- Immobilize and elevate the bitten extremity so that it is at the same level as the heart. Don't apply pressure.
- Treatment with antivenin should only occur in the hospital.
- Snake bite treatment has been plagued over the years with poor suggestions and bad information. The following is a list of things to avoid because they are either harmful to the patient or just do not work:
  - The Sawyer Extractor™
  - Avoid pressure immobilization. Simple immobilization is fine, but has no proven benefit.
  - Electrotherapy should not be used and can be harmful.
  - Do not use ice as it may worsen local tissue damage.
  - Do not attempt to try to catch or kill the offending snake. The recommendations for treating North American snakes' envenomation are the same for all types of snakes. Any attempts to capture the snake may result in additional envenomation and potentially another victim. Even a dead snake's jaw can clamp down and envenomate.
  - Do not use aspirin, as it may worsen bleeding.
  - Do not cut and suck on the wound as it may infect the wound with oral bacteria and it is ineffective at removing venom.
  - Do not use alcohol on the wound or as an oral analgesic.
  - Do not use a tight-fitting tourniquet that restricts blood flow.

Evacuation Guidelines
- Victims of a pit viper bite should be promptly evacuated.

Coral Snake

Background
- Coral snakes in the U.S. have a very distinct color banding pattern.
- An easy way to remember the banding of the deadly coral snake is, "Red on black, venom lack; red on yellow, kill a fellow." This means that a red band next to a yellow (not black) band means danger.
- The bite of the coral snake typically involves a finger, toe, or fold of skin as its jaws are unable to open wide.
- Coral snake venom is more potent than pit viper venom; however, envenomation usually takes up to twelve hours for a full effect.

Symptoms of coral snake envenomation
- Mild, transient pain at the time of the bite
- No local swelling
- Fang marks may be difficult to identify
- Symptoms will often progress rapidly once they appear
- Nausea and vomiting
- Headache
- Abdominal pain
- Sweating and pale skin
- Numbness and abnormal sensations
- Drowsiness
- Euphoria
- Respiratory difficulties

Treatment
- Treatment and evacuation principles are the same as for envenomation with a pit viper.

Evacuation Guidelines
- Victims of a coral snake bite should be promptly evacuated.

Snakes Worldwide

- Worldwide, it is estimated there are a minimum of 1 to 2 million annual snakebite "incidences". This number includes bites by non-venomous species.
- Of that number, roughly 50,000 to 100,000 bites result in fatalities worldwide. Many of the world's most venomous snakes have venoms that are very straightforward and 'easy' to treat effectively with the proper anti venoms.
- There are some that cause a clinical explosion of problems for which anti venoms are not very effective.
- Following is a list of the most dangerous and deadly snakes in the world using the potency of snake's venom, fatalities, and aggressiveness into account.
- These bites must be treated aggressively, so it is essential to get to help quickly.
- Pressure dressings and tourniquets are appropriate. Anti venom should be administered as soon as possible so immediate evacuation is essential.
- It is important to know where these deadly snakes are found and to be aware of appropriate treatments and where hospitals would be located as a traveler goes to these various countries.

Black Mamba: The black mamba is found throughout most countries in Sub-Saharan Africa and is incredibly fast, traveling at speeds of up to 12 miles per hour. The Black Mamba is aggressive and territorial, characteristics not usually attributed to snakes. This snake is usually found in an olive green color – it's the inside of its mouth that is black. Its poison is a very fast acting neuro-toxin.

Russell Viper: This snake is found in Asia, throughout the Indian subcontinent, much of Southeast Asia, southern China and Taiwan. It is responsible for more human fatalities than any other venomous snake. It is a member of the big four venomous snakes in India, which are together responsible for nearly all Indian snakebite fatalities.

Egyptian Cobra: This is the most common cobra in Africa and is responsible for many deaths there. It typically makes its home in dry to moist savanna and semi-desert regions, with at least some water and vegetation.

Mozambique spitting cobra: This is a type of cobra, native to Africa. It is considered one of the most dangerous snakes in Africa, second only to the Mamba. It can spit its venom.

Australian brown snake: This is a deadly Australian snake. 1/14,000 of an ounce of this venom is enough to kill a person. It is the world's second most venomous land snake. Brown Snakes are very fast moving and highly aggressive. When agitated, they will hold their necks high, appearing in a somewhat upright S-shape. The snake will occasionally chase an aggressor and strike at it repeatedly.

Death Adder: This snake is native to Australia. It is one of the most venomous land snakes in Australia and the world.

Mosquitos

Prevention

- Mosquitoes transmit many deadly diseases
- Mosquitoes are most active at dusk, so staying indoors during that time will decrease contact.
- Choose a campsite that is high and away from standing water.
- Wear clothing with long sleeves and long socks with the pants tucked into the socks or boots.
- Wear clothing that is tightly woven, such as nylon, and is loose fitting so that a mosquito cannot bite through the clothing.
- Wear insect repellant on uncovered skin.
- DEET is the gold standard for insect repellants.
    - It is sold in formulations of 5%-35%.
    - Use formulations of 10% or less in children and avoid use altogether in infants under 6 months
    - Use formulations of 30% to 35% in malaria-prone areas on adults.
    - Do not use sunscreens that contain DEET as sunscreens need to be used liberally and often, whereas DEET should be used less often.
    - When using both sunscreen and DEET, apply the sunscreen first then apply the DEET approximately 30 minutes later.
    - DEET may be applied to clothing but should be washed off as soon as repellent is no longer needed.
    - Oil of Lemon Eucalyptus is a plant-based substance and Picaridin (a chemical known also as Icaradin) are shown to be as effective as low concentrations of DEET in repelling mosquitoes. They have a pleasant fragrance and sprays containing these are far less likely to irritate the skin than DEET repellents.
- Permethrin is a naturally occurring compound with insecticidal and repellent properties that will stay on the material for weeks when properly applied.
- Apply permethrin to clothing and bedding, especially mosquito netting. Do not apply directly to skin.
- If you are traveling to a location where you are unsure of the mosquito risk you can consult the CDC website: http://www.cdc.gov/travel/index.htm
- In summary, Permethrin-treated clothing plus DEET repellent confers the best protection.

Spiders

Background

- Many spiders are venomous, but only a few of them are dangerous to humans.
  - Many spiders do not have enough venom to affect a human.
  - Many spiders do not have fangs large enough to penetrate human skin.
- Dangerous North American spiders include the black widow, brown recluse, and hobo spider.

Black Widow

Background
- The black widow is a female of the Lactrodectus species that is found worldwide.
- It is characterized by black shiny skin and a red mark on the belly (often an hour-glass shape).
- They make their homes in irregular webs in sheltered corners of vineyards, fields, and gardens. They can also be found under stones, logs, vegetation, and trash heaps.

Symptoms of a black widow bite
- A sharp pin prick is usually felt, although not always.
- Faint red bite marks may appear later.
- Muscle stiffness and cramps of the bitten limb may develop and will typically spread to involve the abdomen and chest.
- Additional symptoms include headache, chills, fever, heavy sweating, dizziness, nausea, vomiting, and severe abdominal pain.
- These symptoms occur within 30-60 minutes of the bite.
- Most black widow bites have excellent long-term outcomes.
- Short-term problems include high blood pressure, altered mental status, and abdominal pain.
- One study showed that only 25% of bite victims will go on to have the more serious symptoms. Very few humans die from black widow bites.

Treatment
- Catch the spider, if possible, as even a smashed spider can be identified under the microscope of an experienced entomologist.
- Clean the bite with soap and water.
- Relieve pain with a cold compress and oral medications. Cold compresses will also reduce circulation to help slow the spread of the venom.

Evacuation Guidelines
- The victim of a bite should be evacuated as soon as possible as envenomation can become very painful, and the patient may warrant more serious medical attention than can be given in the wilderness.

Brown Recluse

Background
- Loxosceles reclusa or the brown recluse is most commonly found in the southern states and up the Mississippi River Valley as far north as Wisconsin.
- The brown recluse is nondescript and brown, although some will have a violin-shaped marking on the top front body portion.
- Its habitat includes small sticky webs under rocks and woodpiles. The brown recluse also likes warm human habitats including homes, warehouses, and sheds.

Symptoms of a brown recluse bite
- The initial bite is usually painless. The victim is unaware that a bite even occurred until it becomes painful, red, itchy, and swollen two to eight hours after the bite.
- The majority of bites remain localized, healing within three weeks without serious complication or medical intervention.
- Additional symptoms include fever, weakness, vomiting, joint pain, and rash.
- In more serious cases, the bite may cause significant local tissue damage, manifested in the following ways:
    - It will have a white core surrounded by an erythematous patch of skin ending in a white, blue border. This can resemble a "bulls-eye" pattern.
    - Within 24-48 hours, the central core will blister if the envenomation is more serious. This central core may continue to expand over a period of days to weeks if it is a more serious envenomation. Damage to the patient's skin and subcutaneous fat may occur leading to ulcerations.

Treatment
- Catch the spider, if possible, to allow for identification.
- Cleanse the bite with soap and water.
- Elevate the extremity and loosely immobilize it.
- Place a cold compress and give oral analgesics for pain control.
- The patient is in no immediate danger unless systemic signs begin appearing such as large patches of inflammation or blood in the urine.
- Hospital management is only necessary if systemic symptoms occur.

Evacuation Guidelines
- There is no need to evacuate the patient unless they develop systemic symptoms.

Ticks

Background
- Ticks transmit many diseases including Lyme Disease, Rocky Mountain spotted fever, and Colorado tick fever. Only the mosquito transmits more diseases worldwide than the tick.
- Ticks are found in areas replete with weeds, shrubs, and trails.
- They will often be found at forest boundaries where deer and other mammals reside.
- Ticks will sit on whatever low-hanging shrub it can find with arms outstretched.
- Once on a person, they may then take up to several hours to find a suitable spot to attach.
- A tick will then feed on the blood of the host for an average of two to five days.

Prevention
- Check clothing and exposed skin for ticks twice daily.
- Tuck shirts into pants and pants into socks.
- Wear smooth, close-woven, loose-fitting clothing.
- Soak or spray clothing with Permethrin.
- Wear DEET insect repellent.

Treatment
- When a tick is removed in less than 48 hours patients rarely get Lyme disease. For this reason it is very important to check for ticks often and to remove them immediately upon discovery.
- Tick removal:
    - Use thin-tipped tweezers or forceps to grasp the tick as close to the skin surface as possible.
    - Pull the tick straight upward with steady even pressure.
    - Wash the bite with soap and water, then wash hands after the tick has been removed.

- Watch for local infection and symptoms of tick-borne illness (3-30 days), especially headache, fever, and rash.
- The **"DO NOTS"** of tick removal are the following:
    o Do not use petroleum jelly.
    o Do not use fingernail polish.
    o Do not use rubbing alcohol.
    o Do not use a hot match.
    o Do not use gasoline.
    o Do not grab the rear end of the tick. This expels contents and increases the chances of infection.
    o Do not twist or jerk, as this will most likely cause incomplete removal of the tick.

Evacuation Guidelines

- Most patients with tick bites do not require evacuation, especially if the tick is removed within 24-48 hours.
- However, if the patient develops fever, headache, vomiting, rash, or is otherwise ill, the patient should be urgently evacuated.

Hymenoptera (Bees, Wasps and Ants)

Background

- Hymenoptera is the order of insects that includes ants, bees, and wasps.
- Although there is great concern over snake bites, many more people die in the United States from bee, hornet, and wasp stings than from snake bites.
- One sting to an allergic person can be fatal in minutes to hours.
- Non-allergic victims may experience fatal toxicity if they sustain multiple stings.
- It takes between 500-1400 simultaneous stings to cause death by toxicity in the non-allergic patient.
- Multiple stings have become more of a concern in the U.S. since the Africanized Honey Bees ("Killer Bees") first arrived in 1990.

Symptoms of hymenoptera sting

- The local reaction is the most common reaction. It consists of a small red patch that burns and itches with some pain.
- The generalized reaction consists of hives, swelling of lips and tongue, wheezing, abdominal cramps and diarrhea.
- Stings to the mouth and throat are more serious as they may cause airway swelling.
- Victims of multiple stings often experience vomiting, diarrhea, shortness of breath, lightheadedness and may even loss consciousness.

Prevention

- Do not wear any sweet-smelling fragrances often found in after-shaves and perfume. These often attract bees and other insects.
- Bees and wasps are attracted by rotten fruit and fruit syrups.
- Frequent cleaning of garbage areas and proper disposal of old fruit will decrease hymenoptera attraction.
- If an adult has had a full-fledged anaphylactic reaction, they should see an allergist for desensitization.
- A hymenoptera allergic patient should wear medical tags and carry an EpiPen® or equivalent device.

Treatment

- Scrape away the stinger in a horizontal fashion as it may continue to pump toxin into the wound.
  - Try not to grasp the stinger sac as that may pump more venom into the site.
  - However, if one is unable to remove the stinger in a horizontal fashion, removing it any way possible is more important rather than waiting.
- Wash the site with soap and water.
- Place a cold compress or ice on the site. This can ease the pain and swelling.
- Give oral pain medication as needed for pain relief.
- Seek immediate advanced medical attention if there is any shortness of breath, wheezing or other breathing concerns.

Scorpions

Background

- Scorpions are found in desert and semiarid climates between 50 degrees north and south latitude.
- Most scorpion stings are not lethal.
- Most scorpion stings result in only local pain and inflammation.
- In the U.S., the medically important scorpion is the Centruroides exilicauda or bark scorpion. This is found in the Southwestern U.S., primarily Arizona and New Mexico. The bark scorpion is long and slender and has a straw-colored yellow appearance with longitudinal stripes.
- In North America, more serious scorpion stings occur in Mexico.
- The bark scorpion can be lethal to infants and the elderly.
- The bark scorpion can be found under wood piles, stumps, firewood piles, trees, and in a moist indoor environment under blankets, clothing, and in shoes.

Symptoms of scorpion sting

- Scorpions may sting multiple times.
- Except for the bark scorpion, most sting symptoms are similar to hymenoptera stings.
- For the bark scorpion, the following conditions apply:
  - The sting causes local pain followed with numbness and tingling.
  - A toxin released at the time of the sting can cause muscle spasms and possibly changes in blood pressure and heart rate.
  - Symptoms include paralysis, muscle spasms, breathing problems, vision problems, swallowing difficulty, and slurred speech.

Prevention

- Check for scorpions in clothing and shake out shoes in areas where the scorpions are prevalent.
- Do not place your hands or feet into unknown areas that you cannot look directly into.

Treatment

- Clean the sting site with soap and water.
- Place a cool compress for pain and swelling. Cooling the wound will facilitate your body's breakdown of the venom and reduce overall pain.
- Oral pain medications can also be given if the patient does not have trouble breathing and the mental status is normal.
- If the scorpion is identified as not being a bark scorpion, treat the sting as follows:
  - Local treatment and monitoring similar to hymenoptera sting is all that is required.
  - Evacuation is not mandated unless the patient develops significant symptoms.

- If the scorpion is identified as a bark scorpion, treat the sting as follows:
    - Evacuate as soon as possible as the patient may decompensate rapidly.
    - The need for evacuation is more significant in children and the elderly.

Questions

1. **True or False: When you encounter a black bear you should immediately get into the fetal position and protect your neck.**

2. **True or False: When confronted by a cougar you should face it and appear very noisy as if you are a threat to it.**

3. **True or False: Once a snake has been killed, there is little risk in picking up a snake—in fact it is encouraged for identification.**

4. **Which one of the following is an appropriate tick-removal technique?**
    a. Light a match and burn the rear end of the tick
    b. Lather the tick and surrounding skin with Vaseline to require the tick to come up for air
    c. Remove gently with tweezers grasping as close to the skin as possible and pulling straight out
    d. Using tweezers, twist the tick so it will disengage its mouth and then pull straight out

5. **Which one of the following is an appropriate field first aid measure for snake bite wound care?**
    a. Cut down the track of the bite with a clean knife and suck on the cut
    b. Give aspirin for the pain
    c. Give antivenin early in the field if you have some in your aid kit
    d. Immobilize the bite at the level of the heart and require the patient to rest

6. **True or False: The stinger from a honeybee should be removed to prevent further toxin seepage, but one should not try to grasp the venom sack as that might pump more toxin into the wound site.**

7. **A bite from which spider would be cause for immediate evacuation?**
    a. Black widow
    b. Brown recluse
    c. Daddy long legs
    d. Hobo spider
    e. Tarantula

8. **True or False: Most scorpion stings are poisonous and require immediate evacuation.**

ANSWERS
1. f 2. t 3. f 4. c 5. d 6. t 7. a 8. f

CHAPTER 15
Evacuation Guidelines

Objectives:
- Identify important conditions that might require evacuations
- Recognize signs, symptoms, and conditions that require evacuation

Case 15.1

While on a floating trip on the Warm River in Ashton, Idaho, you come to your drop-off spot to see a group of people surrounding a woman who is in distress. She is lying on the ground and is gasping for air and the breaths she can take make a wheezing sound. You suspect she has eaten a local "wild" berry and perhaps is having a reaction to it. What should you do next?

Case 15.2

While hiking, you come upon a man who is resting on the side of the trail with a grimace on his face. He claims that his stomach is hurting but he does not know why. What are some questions you should ask him to help you decide when to evacuate him? What findings would alert you to evacuate this person?

Background

- Determining when to evacuate a patient is one of the biggest and most important decisions in wilderness life support.
- In reality, the decision to evacuate a patient is based on a whole variety of factors:
  o The length of the evacuation
  o The risk to the patient and to the rescuer
  o The necessity of the evacuation
- Some people need to be evacuated for simple injuries such as a foot blister on a hiker.
- Others are based on the critical nature of the condition, such anaphylaxis.
- Others are based on the patient's ability to eat.
- Some are based on whether or not their condition is likely to become worse.

Abdominal Problems
- When patients receive serious abdominal injuries, they need to be evacuated immediately.
- General evacuation guidelines:
  o Blood appears in the vomit, feces, or urine
  o The pain is associated with the signs and symptoms of shock
  o The pain persists for longer than 24 hours
  o The pain is localized and there is guarding, rigidity, and tenderness
  o The pain is associated with a fever greater than 102°F
  o The pain is associated with pregnancy
  o The patient is unable to drink or eat

Allergy Problems
- Patients treated for anaphylaxis should be evacuated for further medical evaluation.

Burns
- In the wilderness, the rule of thumb is that a full thickness (third degree) burn that is less than 1% of the TBSA can be treated in the wilderness with proper burn management. This excludes deep burns of the face, hands, feet and genitals. Severe burns greater than 1% should be evacuated.
- In addition, a major burn that meets the following criteria should be evacuated:
    - Partial thickness (second degree) burns greater than 10% of the TBSA
    - Major burns of the hand, face, feet, or genitals
    - Burns with inhalation injury
    - Electric burns
    - Burns in medically ill patients

Chest Pain
- Patients with suspected heart attack should be evacuated promptly.
- Patients with no clear reason for their chest pain should be strongly considered for evacuation

Diabetic Emergencies
- Hyperglycemic patients should be evacuated if treatment is not working.
- Hypoglycemic patients should be evaluated for evacuation based on effectiveness of treatment and the patient's wishes.

Dislocations
- Due to the possibility of underlying damage, all dislocations should be evacuated and receive further medical evaluation.
- Evacuation may not be necessary for dislocation of the fingers or for chronic dislocations if the patient still has use of the joint after reduction.

Fractures
- Evacuate any patient with suspected fractures.
- Prompt evacuation is necessary with open fractures, fractures of the pelvis or femur, or fractures with decreased motion further from the injury.

Heat-Related Problems
- Any patient treated for heat stroke should be evacuated.
- Recovery from heat cramps or mild heat exhaustion does not necessitate evacuation.

Hypothermia and Frostbite
- A patient fully recovered from mild hypothermia does not require evacuation.
- Patients with moderate and severe hypothermia should be quickly and carefully evacuated.
- Evacuate any patient with frostbite.

Lightning
- Any person involved in a lightning strike should be evacuated.

Neurologic Emergencies
- Evacuate any patient suffering a stroke or who has experienced a seizure.
- A significant change in mental status should lead to patient evacuation.

Pulmonary
- Patients treated for medical emergencies that involve difficulty breathing should be evacuated immediately.
- Patients with mild asthma or hyperventilation syndrome that is successfully treated do not need to be evacuated.

Submersion
- Patients involved in accidental submersion, especially if they lost consciousness, required resuscitation, have difficulty breathing, or have a history of lung disease, need to receive further evaluation in a medical setting.
- Immediate evacuation is necessary for a patient who remains unconscious following a submersion incident.

Wounds
- Evacuation should be prompt when there is a high probability of infection or deep wounds.
- Shock from blood loss that is not reversed by treatment should be quickly evacuated.

Questions

1. While on a campout, a friend of yours falls into the campfire and sustains a burn on his right hand. The burn appears to be deep enough to be considered a third degree burn but occurred only on his right palm and the palmar surface of his fifth finger (pinky), which you estimate to be less than 1% of his TBSA. What is the recommendation for evacuation in this situation?
    a. He can be treated with a wilderness medicine burn kit because his burn occurred over less than 1% of his body area.
    b. He should be evacuated and taken to a hospital for treatment.
    c. With rest, water, and some Neosporin he should be fine.
    d. Wrap the wound for now and if it becomes worse within the next 24-48 hrs, evacuate.

2. Which of the following is NOT a situation where a patient needs to be evacuated due to an abdominal injury?
    a. Blood appears in the vomit, feces or urine
    b. The pain localizes and is there is guarding, rigidity, and tenderness
    c. The pain persists for longer than 24 hours
    d. The patient has watery diarrhea

3. You are on a backpacking trip in the Uintas when a man in your group faints and falls to the ground. You and a friend perform MARCH and begin CPR. He is resuscitated after the first attempt. He did not sustain any injuries from falling to the ground and states afterward that he feels okay to continue with the hike; he just needs to rest a few hours. What is the proper course of action in this case?
    a. Evacuate him immediately and seek medical attention.
    b. Evacuate him immediately, and have him stay home resting or close to a hospital for 24 hours.
    c. Have him rest for four hours, then continue the hike but at a much slower pace.
    d. Continue the hike, but at a much slower pace.

4. While biking in Moab, a friend falls from his bike and dislocates his shoulder. One of the people in your group is a physical therapist and relocates his shoulder. After the successful relocation, your friend is able to move his shoulder. Your friend says that this happens to him all the time. What should be done next?
    a. Attempt to re-dislocate his shoulder and reset it several times. This should help prevent future dislocations.
    b. Do not let him ride anymore. Finish your riding and if possible, evacuate your friend.
    c. Evacuate him immediately and seek medical attention.
    d. If he does not have further problems with his shoulder, he does not need to be evacuated.

5. You are on a day hike when a friend of yours forgot to bring enough water. After a few hours, he begins to act confused and complains of dizziness and fatigue. You give him some of your water and he is still a bit dizzy, but he does not appear to be confused anymore, just a bit fatigued. What should be done next?
    a. Let him keep your water bottle and finish up your hike.
    b. You should rest for a few hours to allow him to drink, then continue your hike.
    c. Evacuate him immediately.
    d. Have him run up the trail for a bit to reset his fluid levels and wake himself up.

ANSWERS
1. b 2. d 3. a 4. d 5. c

CHAPTER 16
Wilderness Medical Kits

Bringing appropriate medical equipment and supplies into the backcountry is essential. This chapter discusses general considerations, planning and preparation, and specific items that can be used for multiple purposes.

General Considerations

- The decision of what equipment to bring depends on multiple aspects of a specific trip: type of activity, group size, distance, and time and availability of evacuation. For example, a backpacking trip of seven days over high, mountainous terrain far from civilization requires a medical kit that is lightweight and contains items that can treat emergencies related to high-altitude illness, cold exposure, trauma, geographically specific infectious diseases, and avalanches. This is in contrast to a one-day river trip near a highway where weight is less of an issue and evacuation may be aided by a nearby vehicle. In the latter scenario, a kit with supplies to treat emergencies related to water sports, cold exposure, and trauma would be appropriate.

- While having the right equipment is important, it is impossible to carry all foreseeable items into the backcountry. Improvising with what is available becomes necessary for any trip. Items that are versatile or those brought for other purposes such as safety pins, gauze, duct tape, and camping equipment can be used in various ways and can replace specific items.

- When in a group and especially if you are the medical leader, you need to consider the age, past medical history, and allergies of each member of the group. In addition, everyone should have a kit containing personal medications. The main kit can also be divided among the group.

- Keep in mind that people have allergies to medicines and tapes, so bring alternative medicines and supplies.

- Several options exist for types of kits. The two most important aspects are protection of the supplies from the elements and organization of the equipment. Cordura is an excellent material for most activities except water-related activities where a waterproof container is necessary. Be careful of the medications that need to be at a certain temperature to maintain their integrity.

- Many commercial kits are available and carry essential supplies and equipment but do not contain prescription medications. Making your own kit is another option and can save money. Either way, you will need to make adjustments and bring items that pertain to the specific activity.

Specific Items

Though it is not practical to list each item that should be placed in every type of medical kit, some general items as well as specific items are listed below. The acronym PAWS, as outlined below, is a way to remember a general guideline of items to place in a kit.

P - Prevention / Procedures

Prevention can make or break a trip and good judgment is the key ingredient. Many crisis situations can be avoided with adequate planning and preparation.

Water filter	Purification tablets	Gloves	Sun screen	Soap
Blister prevention	Insect repellant and barriers	Immunizations for specific destinations	Oral rehydration packets	Extra food and clothing

Procedures require certain tools that may be used in a wide variety of situations. Items in boldface are recommended for a basic kit, while the remainder should be considered for longer trips.

Needles (two to three sizes)	Zerowet® for wound irrigation	Syringes for wound irrigation	SAM splint/ finger splints
Dental wax – filling	Ziploc® bags	Scissors	Safety Pins
Headlamp	Tongue depressors	Splinter removal forceps	

A - Analgesics / Antibiotics / Antiseptics

This category comprises medications and other substances for a wide variety of uses in the backcountry. Each member of the group should bring his or her own medications for any preexisting medical problems.

- Over the counter acetaminophen and NSAIDs are the strongest analgesics (pain control medications) that the wilderness life support provider should use.
- Antibiotics are beyond the scope for wilderness life support

Acetaminophen (Tylenol)	Ibuprofen (Motrin)	Diphenhydramine (Benadryl)	Aloe Vera
Epinephrine (EpiPen)	Glucose paste	Simethicone (Mylanta)	Aspirin

W - Wound Care

This is by far the area that will get the most use, as most injuries are simple wounds. Bring plenty for the small wounds. A wound requiring daily dressings can quickly exhaust a kit's supplies on extended trips.

Gloves	Wound closure strips	Tincture of benzoin	Alcohol swabs
Band-Aids®	2nd Skin®	Large trauma dressing	4x4" gauze
Irrigation equipment	Gauze wrap	Antiseptic towelettes	Antibiotic ointment
Sterile scrub brush	Sterile dressing	Tape (cloth/duct)	Elastic bandage (ACE®)
Q-tip®	Eye pad	Triangular bandage	

S - Survival

The potential for the group members to be separated and other worst-case scenarios need to be considered. Below is a table of items each group member should have on his or her person.

ID/pencil/notepad	Flashlight	Map/compass	Matches, lighter
Knife/multi-tool	Nylon cord	Bandana/ace wrap	Energy bar
Gauze/tape	Whistle/mirror	Medications	Space blanket

Other Medical Kits

As each trip varies according to duration and type of activity, the kit should be tailored accordingly. Below are a few items that one should bring for a specific trip or situation.

In-vehicle Medical Kit

A medical kit to keep in the car can serve as an extra kit while traveling to a trailhead and as a more comprehensive kit in the event of an evacuation. This kit comprises the previously listed items in addition to any of the following:

Ropes, rescue equipment	Splints, traction equipment	Board for spinal immobilization (folding or short)	Foil or window shelter
Blankets	Extra food, water	Scissors	Flashlight
Battery cables	Long-burning candles	Lighter, matches	Toilet paper
Radio, citizens band	Tarp	Saw, metal cutting	Chains
Fire extinguisher	Flares (6)	Shovel	Cables/tow chain
Wedge block	Stove, cookware	Large burn dressings	Additional gloves

Specific Activities

Specific activities or certain patient populations may need other equipment in addition to those items listed above:

Climbing and Canyoneering
- Bring rescue equipment for difficult evacuation, including extra splints, wound care supplies, and water purification.

Mountaineering
- Bring high-altitude items such as extra sunglasses, ophthalmic medications, avalanche safety and rescue equipment. Also, bring cold-exposure materials such as hand and foot warmers, space blanket, and aloe vera (frostbite).

Water sports
- Bring rescue devices depending on the depth of water.

Pediatric
- Bring medications in chewable or suspension form with the appropriate dosing according to weight. Smaller sizes of equipment may also be necessary.

Questions

1. **What are the four elements of the acronym PAWS?**
    a. Prevention/Procedures, Analgesics/Antibacterials/Antiseptics, Wound care, Survival
    b. Pulmonary, Aortic, Water, Septic
    c. Pills, Airway, Water, Solids
    d. Pyretics, Anti-inflammatories, Wool, Shovel

2. **What are some examples of items to pack into a medical kit that would help prevent an emergency?**
    a. Road flare
    b. Shampoo
    c. Water filter
    d. Novel

3. **What is the main concern with performing a closure of an open wound while in the wilderness?**
    a. Pain
    b. Infection
    c. Non-aesthetic scar
    d. Re-injury

4. **Seeing how you cannot carry all items used to treat every foreseeable illness, at times you have to use items that are versatile and can be used to improvise. Which of the following is a list of good examples?**
    a. Duct tape, gauze bandage, safety pins
    b. Portable gurney, surgical scissors, 5L water jug
    c. IV solution, medical splint, 2-pint alcohol bottle

ANSWERS
1. a 2. c 3. b 4. a

CHAPTER 17

Water Disinfection and Hydration

Objectives:
- Describe various waterborne pathogens that may cause illness from contaminated water.
- Describe three pre-disinfection techniques to initiate the water purification process.
- Describe limitations and techniques for water disinfection through the use of heat, filtration, and halogenation.
- Understand the concept of basic hygiene as it relates to minimizing gastrointestinal illness.

> ## Case 17.1
>
> A group of backpackers traverse a difficult ridge in the High Uinta Wilderness. On reaching the other side they are exhausted and thirsty. Having consumed all available water, they search for the nearest stream.
>
> The icy cold waters are reasonably clear, so they fill their canteens and hydration bladders. As one of the most lightweight options, iodine and chlorine tablets were brought for water disinfection. Although very thirsty, the backpackers are careful to follow the directions on the packaging before drinking the water. The remainder of the trip is uneventful.
>
> About seven days later, two of the hikers develop gastrointestinal distress. They both complain of abdominal cramping and watery diarrhea. One of them develops a low-grade fever of 100.1°F, yet her symptoms resolve over the next few days. The other hiker is more symptomatic with nausea, vomiting, and weight loss. After several days, he is admitted to the hospital because of dehydration and requires IV fluid resuscitation.
>
> During his evaluation, fecal specimens reveal microscopic oocysts, but no white blood cells. There are no other specific signs or symptoms. An infectious disease physician orders some specialized tests, which confirm an infection with Cryptosporidium.

Background

The human body depends on a constant influx of water for survival. Gastrointestinal illness from poorly treated water is a major cause of diarrhea and dehydration in the wilderness. In a survey of wilderness hikers seven days into their trip, diarrheal illness was the second most common medical complaint (56%), closely following blisters (64%).

The goal of water decontamination and disinfection is to eliminate or reduce the number of infectious microorganisms to an acceptably low number.

Unfortunately, merely straining water through a handkerchief and then judging water by its taste, appearance, and location are unreliable methods for determining its safety for consumption. By understanding and practicing the guidelines in this chapter, one should be able to minimize the risk of acquiring waterborne illness in the wilderness.

Microbiologic Etiology

Waterborne pathogens fall into four major categories:
- Bacteria
- Viruses
- Protozoa
- Helminths

The likelihood of encountering any of these microorganisms depends on the location and exposure of the water source to contamination.

- Watershed areas with animal grazing and human contact have different risks than water that seemingly comes from an underground source. Some organisms may reside in particular soils and contaminate surface water.

- As a general guideline, pristine watershed areas tend to be free of viral agents. With increasing human and animal contact, viral contamination becomes more of a concern.

- In the field, it can be very difficult to determine who or what has been in the area before you. In order to be safe, one should adhere to the principle that all wilderness water sources are contaminated.

- In the past, much attention has been given to the protozoan *Giardia lamblia* as a cause of wilderness gastrointestinal illness. While it is an important organism to consider, some experts believe it is much more likely that bacteria cause the majority of wilderness gastrointestinal illness in North America.

Pre-Disinfection Techniques

Purification

When water is initially collected, it is important to minimize accumulated particulate matter. Organic and inorganic particles can interfere with the disinfection process, as well as make for an unpleasant drinking experience.

Two of the following steps involve waiting. Depending on the urgency of your situation, you will have to decide if you have enough time and adapt accordingly. It is imperative to understand that these procedures do not disinfect water but enhance the disinfection process and drinking experience.

Screening
This is the process of removing the largest contaminants. This involves using a primary filter as a screen to hold back dirt, plant, and animal matter. Many filtration systems already have a "pre-filter" attached. If one is filling a container by dipping or pouring, he can screen out unwanted debris by pouring the water through a cloth, such as a bandana, handkerchief, or even a t-shirt. One should always include this step in preparations.

Standing
Having the water remain undisturbed for a period of time allows particles that were small enough to pass through the screening material to fall to the bottom of the container. Within as little as one hour, even muddy or turbid water will show significant improvement as the silt settles. After some settling has occurred, the clearer water can be decanted from one container into another, leaving the sediment behind.

Flocculating
This is a method of removing particulate matter that is so small that it would normally stay suspended in water indefinitely. Adding specific chemicals to the water can promote agglomeration of smaller particles until a complex forms that is large enough to precipitate. One such chemical is "alum," which can be purchased from the grocery store. It is also found in baking powder. Add a "pinch" for every gallon of water and then stir it gently for about five minutes. After stirring, allow the water to stand and settle before decanting off the cleaner water. In wilderness settings, the fine, white ashes from burned wood are rich in mineral salts containing some of these flocculating compounds.

Disinfection Methods

Generally speaking you should always try to use two different methods for treating water. There are several choices from which you can choose, depending upon your cirumstances:

Heat

Pathogens, including cysts and eggs, are readily destroyed by heat. The thermal effectiveness for killing pathogens depends on a combination of temperature and exposure time. Because of this, lower temperatures can be effective with longer contact times. Pasteurization applies this science with carefully controlled temperature. Without a thermometer, it is too difficult and risky to gauge temperature short of boiling.

The boiling point of water is 100°C (212°F). At this temperature, disinfection has generally occurred by the time the water boils. This disinfection has occurred due to the fact that water does not necessarily need to be boiling in order to be disinfected. Because it is difficult to determine the exact temperature of the water, boiling is the safest way to ensure that an appropriate temperature has been reached. One important characteristic of boiling points is that they decrease in temperature with increasing elevation. Some physicians believe this does not make an appreciable difference in water disinfection times. However, the CDC recommends boiling water for three minutes if one is located above 6,562 feet (2000 m).

Using heat properly is a very reliable method for water disinfection. Remember to use a pot cover to preserve fuel when heating water. Also, bring the water to a rolling boil to wash back down any pathogens on the inside of the container and assure the surface of the water has reached the boiling point.

Filters

Filters screen out bacteria, protozoa, helminths, and their cysts and eggs, but are not very reliable for eliminating viruses.

Viruses tend to adhere to other particles or clump together, which helps remove some of them by filtration. Nevertheless, they are so small (less than 0.1 micron) that they cannot be eradicated by filters alone. Some filters are impregnated with iodine and bactericidal crystals in an attempt to destroy the viruses as they pass through the material. However, these additions are of questionable efficacy.

Because filters work by trapping small particles in their pore matrix, they clog and become less effective over time. Operating a pump as it becomes clogged can force pathogens through it and contaminate the water.

Interpreting advertised specifications for filters can be tricky. The best way to evaluate a given filter is to ascertain its functional removal rate of various organisms. For example, a filter labeled "effective against pathogens" does not truly describe its efficacy. Filters need to eliminate down to the 0.2 micron range (absolute size, not nominal) to be effective for most pathogens, even though larger pore sizes of 0.3 to 0.4 microns may work for many applications.

For practical usage, filters should only be deployed WITH the addition of another disinfection method, unless in areas where human contact is limited and watershed areas are protected. When uncertain, you should use one of the other methods of disinfection as a final step.

Halogenation

Iodine and chlorine can be very effective as disinfectants against viruses and bacteria. Halogens are typically faster and more convenient than boiling water. However, their effectiveness against helminths and protozoa varies greatly, and they are more costly. *Cryptosporidium* cysts are extremely resistant to halogen disinfection. The amount of halogen required to destroy these is impractical for drinking.

Regardless of this limitation, the major problem with chemical disinfection is that most people do not perform it properly. Disinfection depends on both halogen concentration and contact time. Factors that affect halogen concentration include water temperature, pH and the presence of contaminants. Chlorine is more sensitive to these factors, and is thus less suitable for cold, contaminated water. In these conditions, both halogens require increased contact time and/or concentration. Turbid water should be allowed to settle before halogenation because particulate matter can deactivate the available halogen, rendering disinfection incomplete.

Another challenge with halogens is their unpleasant taste. This can be remedied in several ways, but must be done after disinfection. Ascorbic acid (vitamin C) can reduce some of the poor taste. Flavored drink mixes have the benefits of masking some taste and sometimes containing ascorbic acid. Activated charcoal can also be used to reduce the chemical load after disinfection.

There has been some concern that outdoor enthusiasts might ingest too much iodine over a prolonged period. Some studies have demonstrated changes in thyroid function after prolonged use, although the specific amount of time has not been clearly identified. A general guideline is to avoid using high levels of iodine (recommended tablet doses) for more than one to two months. Persons planning extended use may warrant thyroid function studies before leaving and after returning.

For safety, persons with thyroid disease or who are pregnant should not use iodine. People may develop hypersensitivity reactions to iodine.

Other Methods

Ultraviolet radiation (UVR)

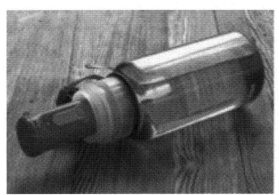

Figure 17.2 Photo by Coronium

UVR has gained popularity as a portable means of water disinfection. Preliminary data show that it can even be effective against the cysts of *Cryptosporidium*. The UV light destroys the DNA of microbes, making them unable to reproduce and cause sickness in humans. Although this method is more expensive, it offers the easiest path to safe water. UVR does have some inherent difficulties, however. It requires a large amount of energy to run a UV lamp and extra batteries are necessary. Additionally, in cold weather, batteries may not be able to provide enough energy to safely power the device. Plus, they are breakable.

Other constraints pertain to water container size and amount of particulate contamination. Water must be clear for UVR use since particulate matter can act as a shield for the pathogens against the UVR.

All factors considered, this method seems more appropriate for urban international settings than for wilderness travel.

Chlorine Dioxide

Chlorine dioxide has shown promising results. It has been around for quite some time, but has recently been made available for consumer water disinfection. There are both liquid and tablet options on the market.

This substance is chemically different from "chlorine." It is much less reactive with pollutants and has a wider range of effective pH. It imparts much less of an offensive taste than halogens. Additionally, it is one of the only chemical disinfectants shown to be useful against *Giardia* and *Cryptosporidium*.

Summary of Treatment Method Efficacy

Infectious Agent	Heat	Filtration	Chemical
Bacteria	+	+	++
Viruses	+	-	+
Protozoa and cysts	++	++	+
Helminths and oocytes	++	++	+

Prevention

Hygiene

As a final note, washing hands and cleaning eating utensils can prevent gastrointestinal illness.

Several studies have shown that hikers are much less likely to develop diarrheal illnesses when they practice proper hygiene. This means using warm, soapy water for cleaning. Being in the great outdoors does not exempt one from hand washing after urination and, particularly, defecation. Eating and cooking utensils should be cleaned thoroughly after each use. Keep your personal utensils out of community cooking gear, and make sure anyone who is sick avoids the food preparation areas.

The same results can theoretically and possibly more easily be accomplished with an alcohol-based hand sanitizer. Remember that hand sanitizer is only effective when there is no visible contamination on your hands. If visible contamination is present, it should be washed away with soap and water if possible.

Questions

1. Which one of the following is considered to be the most likely cause of wilderness gastrointestinal illness in North America?
    a. Bacteria
    b. *Cryptosporidium*
    c. *Giardia lamblia*
    d. Viruses

2. When using heat for water disinfection, the best method incorporates:
    a. Adding iodine or chlorine to boiling water
    b. Boiling water for 10 to 15 minutes
    c. Flocculation of contaminated water
    d. Screening (filtration) of contaminants before heat treatment

3. For an extra margin of safety, the CDC recommends boiling water for three minutes above what elevation?
    a. 3,500 feet
    b. 5,000 feet
    c. 6,500 feet
    d. 10,500 feet

4. Which of the following is the LEAST likely to be found in pristine watershed areas?
    a. *Cryptosporidium*
    b. *E. coli*
    c. *Giardia lamblia*
    d. Viruses

5. Which of the following is not usually removed by filters?
    a. *Ascaris* eggs
    b. Bacteria
    c. *Giardia*
    d. Viruses

6. When choosing a filter, it is important to:
    a. Choose one that includes activated carbon
    b. Find specific information on the functional removal rate of organisms
    c. Have a nominal pore size of 0.2 microns
    d. Make sure it is "effective against *Giardia*"

7. True/False: Filters impregnated with halogens are effective at killing viruses.

8. True/False: Use of iodine is safe for someone with a pre-existing thyroid condition if it is well controlled by medication.

9. Which of the following is the best method for water disinfection:
   a. Boiling water for 1 minute
   b. Chemical halogenation that properly follows directions
   c. Water filtration with a 0.2 micron absolute pore size
   d. The best method depends on the particular location and group size

10. True/False: One can effectively reduce the risk of diarrheal illness in the backcountry by properly cleaning hands after urinating or defecating.

ANSWERS
1. a 2. d 3. c 4. d 5. d 6. b 7. f 8. f 9. d 10. t

Acronyms

Patient Assessment

Scene Survey

1- Scene Safety
2- Mechanism of Injury/ Nature of Illness
3- Body Substance Isolation
4- Triage

A- Alert
V- Verbal
P- Pain
U- Unresponsive

Primary Survey

M- Massive hemorrhage management

A- Airway with cervical spine stabilization

R- Respiratory

C- Circulation

H- Hypothermia/Hyperthermia and Hike vs Helicopter

Secondary Survey

Head to Toe
Areas of major bleeding
- C-Chest
- A-Abdominal/Pelvis
- R-Renal/Retroperitoneal
- T-Thigh
- S-Skin/Street

Assessment of extremities
- C-Circulation
- S-Sensation
- M-Motor Function

Vitals

Time:			
AVPU:			
HR:			
RR:			
SCTM:			
PERRL:			

History

S- Signs/Symptoms
A- Allergies
M- Medications
P- Past Pertinent Hx
L- Last ins/outs
E- Events

C- Character
O- Onset
L- Location
D- Duration
E- Exacerbation
R- Relief
R- Radiation

Plan & Problem List
Subjective/Objective/Assessment/Plan

Cervical Spine Assessment
C- Cervical midline tenderness
S- Sensory and/or motor deficit
P- Pain or psychological distractor
I- Intoxication
N- Neurological deficit
E- Events

Patient with Altered Mental Status
A- Allergies/ Altitude
E- Environment/ Epilepsy
I- Infection
O- Overdose
U- Underdose
T- Trauma
I- Insulin
P- Psychological disorder
S- Stroke

Potential Sources of Major Bleeding: CARTS

CHEST	The chest is a common source of bleeding, particularly in high-energy trauma. Look for shortness of breath, pain with breathing, and coughing up blood. Examine for chest tenderness, crepitance over the ribs and sternum, flail chest and crackling noises of the chest consistent with air under the skin.
ABDOMEN/PELVIS	Assume abdominal and/or pelvis bleeding in every trauma victim until proven otherwise. Look for bruising over the abdomen and pelvis. Palpate for abdominal and pelvic tenderness on compression.
RENAL	Usually the bleeding is from the kidneys. Look for blood in the urine if you have a prolonged time with the victim. Examine for tenderness of the spine and chest and the lowest level of the ribs.
THIGH	This may occur if there is a femur fracture. Look for deformity, swelling and bruising of the thigh. Palpate for tenderness and crepitance of the thigh.
SKIN/STREET	This is the most obvious place for a rescuer to detect blood. A common error in the wilderness setting is the failure to remove clothing or to roll the patient to look for bleeding. Also, ensure that you survey the area immediately surrounding the victim for a large amount of blood on the ground that may have come from the victim. Specifically, an arterial injury that bleeds significantly may be in spasm at the time you are evaluating the victim and not be an obvious source of bleeding.

Glossary of Terms

A

abandonment: To leave a patient in need of medical attention alone or with someone who is not capable of providing care.

abrasion: A type of wound that consists of one or more layers of skin being scraped away.

acclimatization: The process of physiologically adjusting to a new environment, such as a hotter environment or higher altitude.

Achilles tendon: The tendon that connects the muscles of the lower leg to the heel bone.

acute: An immediate problem that is not chronic.

AED: Shorthand for automated external defibrillator.

allergen: Any substance that causes an allergic reaction.

ambulatory: Able to walk.

AMI: Acute myocardial infarction; a sudden heart attack.

amnesia: Loss of memory.

amputation: To cut off a limb or other appendage of the body, especially in a surgical operation.

analgesic: A medication that alleviates pain without loss of consciousness.

anaphylaxis: A sudden severe and potentially fatal allergic reaction in somebody sensitive to a substance, marked by a drop in blood pressure, difficulty in breathing, itching, and swelling.

anesthetic: An agent that produces a partial or complete loss of sensation.

angina pectoris: A medical condition in which lack of blood to the heart causes severe chest pains.

anterior: Front surface.

antibiotic: A substance that prevents growth of or destroys microorganisms.

antidiarrheal: A substance that is used to prevent and treat diarrhea.

anti-emetic: A substance that is used to prevent and treat vomiting.

antihistamine: A drug that is used to counteract the effects of histamines.

anti-inflammatory: A substance used to reduce inflammation.

antipyretic: An agent that reduces or alleviates a fever.

antiseptic: An agent that reduces or prevents infection, especially by eliminating or reducing the growth of microorganisms that cause disease or decay.

antivenin: An antiserum containing antibodies to a specific venom – same thing as antivenom.

antivenom: An antiserum containing antibodies to a specific venom – same thing as antivenin.

aorta: The main artery that carries blood from the left ventricle of the heart travels to the body.

appendicitis: Inflammation of the appendix, causing severe pain.

artery: A vessel that carries blood from the heart to the rest of the body.

asphyxia: A condition caused by an insufficient intake of oxygen.

asthma: A disease of the respiratory system characterized by shortness of breath and wheezing due to swelling of bronchi and their mucous membranes.

AVPU scale: For *Alert, Verbal, Pain, Unresponsive*—a scale for measuring a patient's level of consciousness.

avulsion: The tearing away or separation of part of the body, usually includes a piece of skin left hanging as a flap.

AWLS: Advanced Wilderness Life Support

B

bacteria: Single-cell microorganisms.

Battle's sign: Bruising behind and below the ears, which indicates a fracture to the base of the skull.

BWLS: Basic Wilderness Life Support.

bony crepitation: Sound or feel of broken bone ends grinding against one another.

BVM: Bag valve mask. A patient ventilation device.

C

cardiac arrest: The termination of heart muscle activity.

cardiopulmonary resuscitation (CPR): Artificial respirations and manual chest compressions that help stimulate lung and heart activity.

cardiovascular system: The heart, the blood vessels, and the blood.

carotid artery: A large artery on each side of the neck that supplies blood to the head.

cerebrovascular accident (CVA): Interruption of regular blood flow to a part of the brain which results in a stroke.

cervical vertebrae: The first seven bones pertaining to the spinal column; the neck bones.

CHF: See **congestive heart failure.**

Chief complaint: The principal complaint of a patient. Also CC.

chronic obstructive pulmonary disease (COPD): A collection of diseases sharing the common symptoms of airway obstruction in the small to medium airways, excessive secretions, and/or constriction of the bronchial tubes.

chronic: A condition of slow progression or long duration; not acute.

clavicle: Collarbone.

CNS: For *Central Nervous System*. The brain and spinal cord.

coccyx: The triangular bone at the base of the spinal column, consisting of four fused vertebrae; the tailbone.

COLDERR: For *Character, Onset, Location, Duration, Exacerbation, Relief, Radiation.*

coma: A prolonged state of deep unconsciousness from which the patient cannot be awakened.

comminuted fracture: A fracture where the bone is crushed or splintered.

conduction: Heat that is lost from a warmer object when it comes in contact with a colder object.

congestive heart failure (CHF): A condition in which blood and tissue fluids congest due to the insufficiency of the heart.

conjunctiva: The delicate membrane lining the eyes.

constipation: Infrequent or difficult bowel movements where the feces are hard and dry.

contusion: A bruise.

convection: Heat lost directly into air or water caused by movement.

COPD: See **chronic obstructive pulmonary disease.**

CSM: For *Circulation, Sensation, Motion.*

D

DEET: An insect repellent.

diabetes mellitus: A disease in which the pancreas produces an insufficient amount of insulin or the cells of the body are unresponsive to insulin. Blood sugars are high.

diaphoresis: Profuse sweating.

diarrhea: Frequent passage of unformed, watery bowel movement.

dislocation: The displacement of a body part, especially of a bone from its usual fitting in a joint.

distal: Away from the center.

dysentery: A disease caused by infection of bacteria, marked by severe bacteria that may produce blood and mucus in the stool.

dyspnea: Difficulty in breathing.

E

ecchymosis: Bruising.

ectopic pregnancy: A pregnancy in which the developing fetus implants outside of the womb, usually in a fallopian tube.

edema: Swelling that is caused by a buildup of excess fluid.

embolism: Obstruction of a blood vessel by a clot of blood, a gas bubble, or a foreign substance.

emetics: Causing vomiting.

emesis: Vomit.

envenomation: Poisoning from a venomous bite or sting.

epidermis: The thin outermost layer of the skin.

epigastric: The upper part of the abdomen.

epistaxis: Nosebleed.

esophagus: The passage down which food moves between the throat and the stomach.

evaporation: A process in which something is changed from a liquid to a vapor.

evisceration: A condition in which abdominal contents are exposed and protruding out from an open wound.

exhalation: The act of breathing out.

F

femoral: Relating to the femur.

fibula: Small lower leg bone between the knee and ankle.

flail chest: A condition where multiple ribs are fractured in two or more places, creating a floating section of rib.

fracture: A break in a bone.

frostbite: Localized tissue damage caused by prolonged exposure to freezing conditions.

frostnip: Superficial frostbite.

fx: Shorthand for *fracture*.

G

gastritis: Inflammation of the stomach lining.

gastroenteritis: Stomach and intestinal inflammation.

gingiva: The gum around the roots of the teeth.

glucagon: A hormone that raises the concentration of glucose in the blood.

gluteals: Buttock muscles.

greenstick fracture: A fracture that only extends part way through the bone, usually occurring in children.

guarding: To protect an injured area through muscle tension and/or physical positioning.

H

heat cramps: Painful spasm of major muscles that are being exercised; caused by dehydration in association with electrolyte depletion.

heat exhaustion: Weakness produced by fluid loss from excessive sweating in a hot environment that causes compensatory shock.

heatstroke: a condition caused by prolonged exposure to high temperatures, in which people experience high fever, headaches, hot dry skin, physical exhaustion, and sometimes physical collapse and coma.

hematoma: Pooling of blood in the form of a tumor.

hemorrhage: Bleeding.

hemostasis: Control of blood flow.

histamine: A natural substance released by the immune system in the body which responds to an injury or foreign protein.

humerus: Upper arm bone.

hx: Shorthand for *history*.

I

IM: For *Intramuscular*.

implied consent: When a patient is unconscious, a minor (if a parent or guardian is unavailable to give consent), or for any other reason unable to decide to be treated, it can be legally assumed that he or she would desire treatment if he or she were capable of making the decision.

incision: A smooth-edged cut made in the skin by a sharp edge.

inflammation: Localized changes in tissue size, color, and temperature, as a reaction to injury.

informed consent: The decision a patient makes to be treated after having been informed of the benefits and potential risks of the proposed treatment.

insulin: The hormone produced in the pancreas required to regulate the amount of glucose in the bloodstream.

ischemia: Inadequate blood supply to an organ.

IV: For *Intravenous*.

J

joint: Where two bones are joined.

K

kidney stone: A hard mass formed in the kidneys and excreted through the urinary tract.

L

laceration: A jagged or torn wound in the skin.

lacrimal: Of or relating to tears.

lesion: A region of an organ or tissue that has been damaged or injured.

ligament: Connective tissue that holds bones together.

lumbar vertebrae: Five bones found in the lower spine between the thoracic vertebrae and the sacrum.

M

malaise: A general feeling of discomfort or illness whose exact cause is difficult to diagnose.

metacarpophalangeal joint (MCP): The first joint on the thumb that connects it to the hand.

MI: See **myocardial infarction.**

MOI: For *Mechanism Of Injury*.

myocardial infarction: Death of a portion of the heart muscle resulting from an obstruction of the blood supply to the heart; a heart attack.

myocardium: Heart muscle.

N

nasopharynx: Posterior part of the nose; the part of the pharynx which connects to the nasal cavity above the soft palate.

necrosis: The death of tissue.

negligence: Failure to use proper care that harms another person to whom you owe a duty of care.

NSAID: For *Nonsteroidal anti-inflammatory drug*. A drug administered for inflammation, fever, and pain.

O

open fracture: A fracture over which the skin is torn or cut.

ophthalmic: Of or relating to the eye.

P

palliate: To soothe pain or make feel better.

palpate: To examine by feeling.

paresthesia: Loss of feeling or unusual sensations; "pins and needles."

patella: The kneecap.

pathogen: A microorganism which produces disease.

pathological: Concerning mental or physical disease.

PE: See **pulmonary embolism.**

pedal: Of or relating to the foot.

permethrin: Insect repellent spray applied to clothing primarily to prevent disease; an insecticide.

PERRL: For *Pupils Equal Round and Reactive to Light*.

PFD: For *Personal flotation device*.

pneumonia: Lung infection or inflammation caused by bacterial or viral infection.

pneumothorax: An accumulation of air in the pleural space caused by a tear in the lining of the lung.

polyuria: Excessive production or passage of urine.

postictal: Pertaining to the period following a seizure.

prone: The face-down position.

pulmonary edema: Fluid accumulation in the lungs.

pulmonary embolism: Obstruction of blood flow in a pulmonary artery or arteriole.

puncture: A wound made by the piercing of a pointed object such as knife, bullet, or ice ax.

Q

quadriceps: Thigh muscles of the thigh used to extend the leg.

R

rabies: A contagious and fatal viral infection of the central nervous system transmitted by the bite of an infected mammal.

raccoon eyes: Bruising around the eyes that suggest a skull fracture.

radiation: Heat transmitted by a warm object.

reduction: A return to normal anatomical relationship.

respiratory arrest: Cessation of normal breathing.

rigor mortis: Stiffness that occurs in a dead body.

RLQ: For *Right Lower Quadrant* of the abdomen.

S

sacrum: The five fused bones of vertebrae at the bottom of the spine

SAMPLE: For *Symptoms, Allergies, Medications, Pertinent medical history, Last intake/output, Events.*

scapula: Shoulder blade.

SCTM: For *Skin Color, Temperature, Moisture.*

sepsis: An illness caused by a buildup of toxins and microorganisms in the blood.

septicemia: "Blood poisoning" from too much bacteria or their toxins in the blood.

SOAP: For *Subjective, Objective, Assessment, Plan.*

sprain: A joint injury in which ligaments are stretched or torn.

strain: Stretching or tearing of tendons or muscle fibers.

subcutaneous: Under the skin.

supine: Positioned with the face up.

syncope: Temporary loss of consciousness; fainting.

T

tachycardia: An abnormally rapid heart rate.

tendinitis: Inflammation of a tendon.

tendon: Connective tissue holding muscle to bone.

thermoregulation: Regulation of body core temperature.

thoracic vertebrae: The twelve vertebrae between the cervical vertebrae and the lumbar vertebrae with ribs attached on either side.

thorax: Chest cavity.

TIA: See **transient ischemic attack.**

transient ischemic attack (TIA): A temporary stroke caused by insufficient blood supply to the brain, with signs and symptoms lasting less than twenty-four hours.

triage: A sorting of patients to determine the order of treatment and transport.

tx: Shorthand for treatment.

tympanic membrane: The eardrum.

U

ulcer: An open sore or lesion on skin or mucous membranes caused by a break in the skin.

urushiol: A resinous oil responsible for the irritant properties of poison ivy, poison oak, and poison sumac.

V

vasoconstriction: A narrowing of blood vessels.

vasodilation: A widening of blood vessels.

vein: A vessel that carries blood toward the heart.

vertigo: Dizziness caused by an equilibrium disturbance.

virus: A microorganism that depends on the cells of another organism as a host for replication.

W

WFR: Wilderness First Responder.

WLS: Wilderness Life Support.

X

xiphoid process: The cartilage protuberance at the lower end of the sternum.

Improvised Litters

In the dire situation where a patient needs to be moved or evacuated, it is best to obtain help. However, a situation might arise where a victim needs to be moved without assistance from Search and Rescue teams.

Carries:

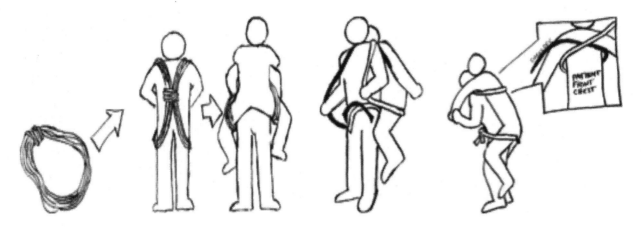

It is possible to carry a victim out using one or two people depending on how many people are available and what material is available.

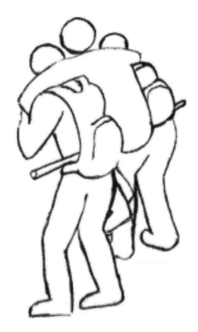

If a litter needs to be created one can be improvised from many different types of objects. Improvisation is the key word. Most flat-surface objects of suitable size can be used as a litter. Such objects include boards, benches, ladders, cots, and poles. If possible, these objects should be padded. Litters can be created by using blankets, ponchos, tents, jackets, shirts, sacks, and bags. Poles can be improvised from branches, tent poles, skis, and other similar items. If poles cannot be found, a large item, such as a blanket, can be rolled from both sides toward the center. Then the rolls can be used to obtain a firm grip to carry the victim. There are literally dozens of ways that people have come up with to create improvised litters. These are a few of them.

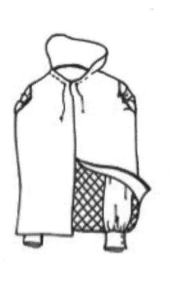
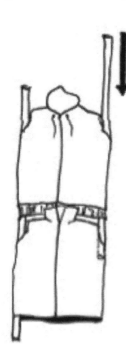

Jacket Litter

If you have at least two jackets or durable long sleeve shirts available, you can easily fashion improvised litters. This is one of the simplest methods of improvised litters, and is very reliable – as long as the jackets are made of a strong material. Fashion improvised litter poles. Button and/or zip two or three jackets. Turn them inside out with their sleeves remaining on the inside. Pass your poles through the sleeves of the jackets.

SOAP NOTE

SUBJECTIVE

OBJECTIVE

LOR:

HR:

RR:

SCTM:

BP:

Pulse:

Temperature:

Symptoms:

Allergies:

Medications:

Past medical history:

Last meal:

Events:

ASSESSMENT

PLAN

Made in the USA
San Bernardino, CA
12 March 2019